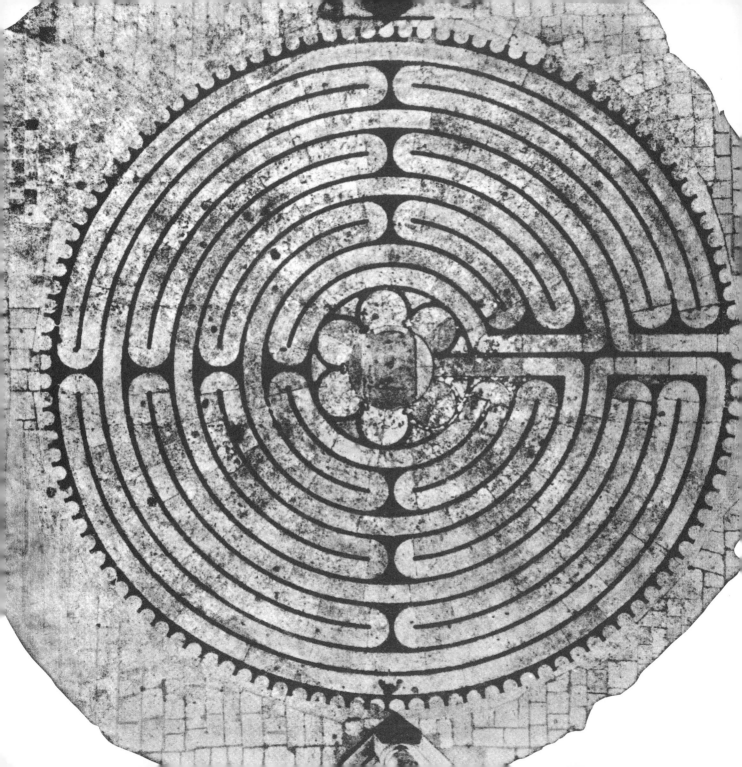

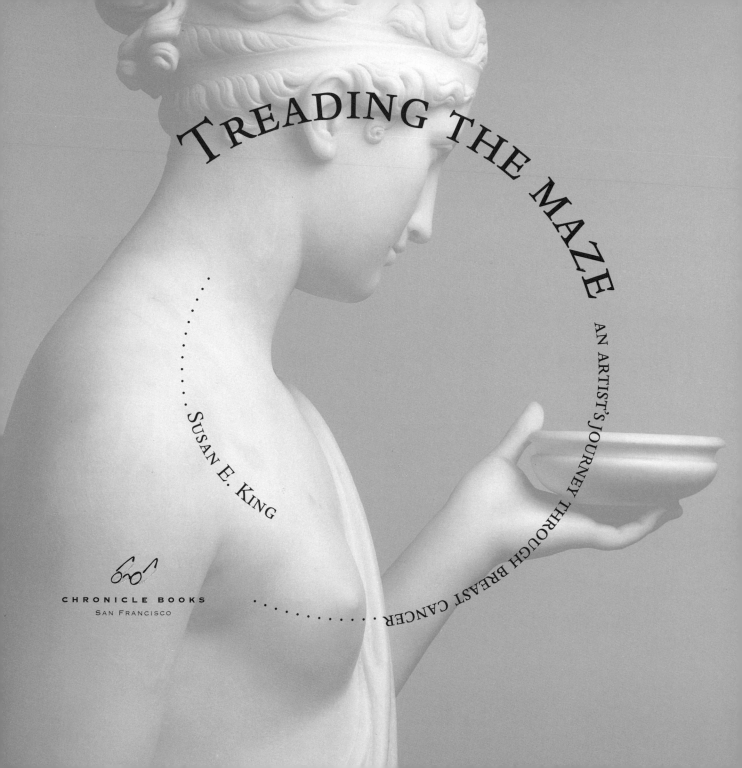

TREADING THE MAZE

AN ARTIST'S JOURNEY THROUGH BREAST CANCER

SUSAN E. KING

CHRONICLE BOOKS
SAN FRANCISCO

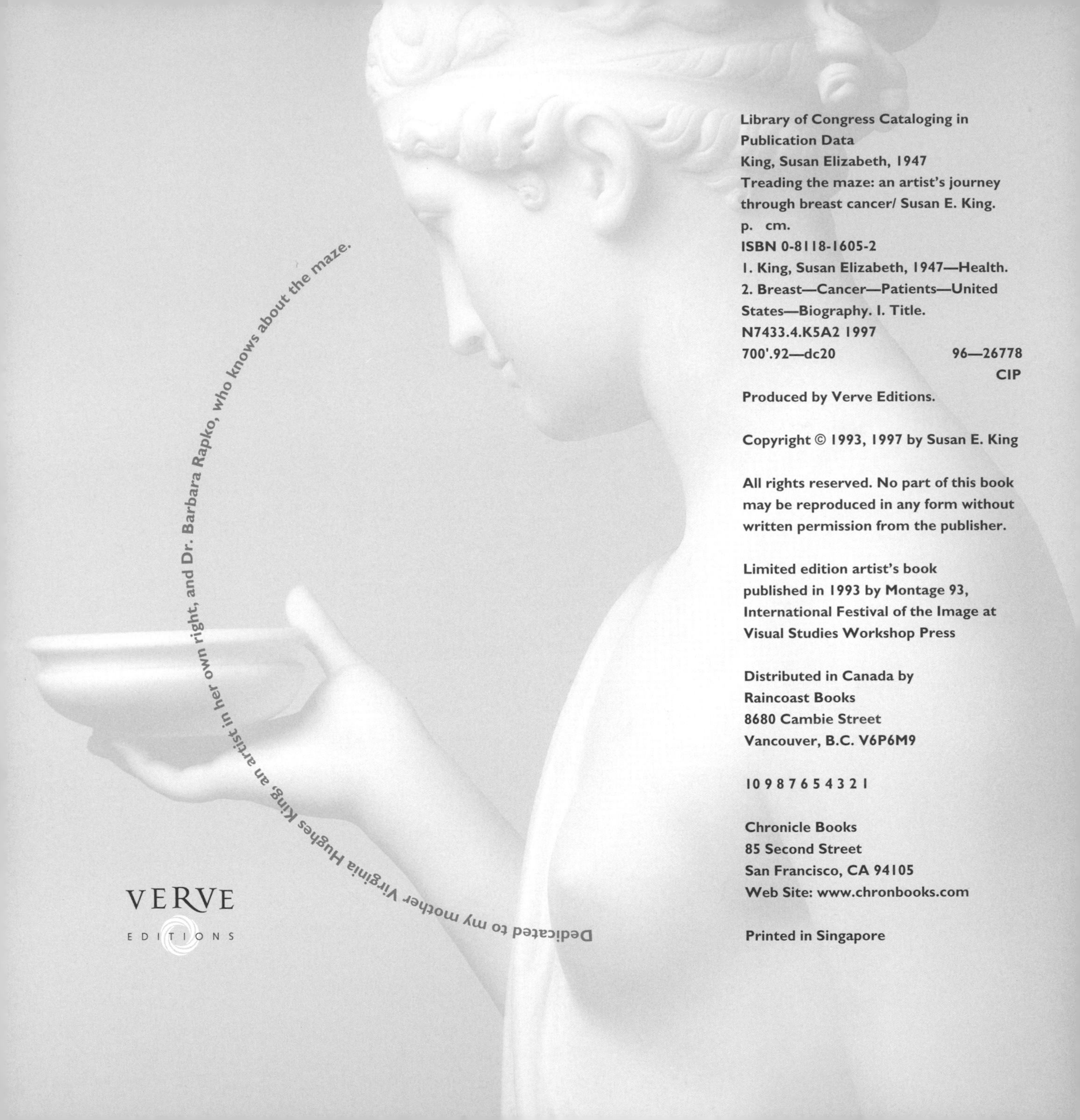

Library of Congress Cataloging in
Publication Data
King, Susan Elizabeth, 1947
Treading the maze: an artist's journey
through breast cancer/ Susan E. King.
p.   cm.
ISBN 0-8118-1605-2
1. King, Susan Elizabeth, 1947—Health.
2. Breast—Cancer—Patients—United
States—Biography. I. Title.
N7433.4.K5A2 1997
700'.92—dc20   96—26778
                                      CIP

Produced by Verve Editions.

Copyright © 1993, 1997 by Susan E. King

Limited edition artist's book
published in 1993 by Montage 93,
International Festival of the Image at
Visual Studies Workshop Press

Distributed in Canada by
Raincoast Books
8680 Cambie Street
Vancouver, B.C. V6P6M9

10 9 8 7 6 5 4 3 2 1

Chronicle Books
85 Second Street
San Francisco, CA 94105
Web Site: www.chronbooks.com

Printed in Singapore

Dedicated to my mother, Virginia Hughes King, an artist in her own right, and Dr. Barbara Rapko, who knows about the maze.

VERVE
EDITIONS

TREADING THE MAZE by Susan King . . . An Artist's Book of Daze Starts Here . . . . "Today the need to travel — especially to places unfamiliar and even unpleasant — motivates much of the art discussed here and can be seen as part of a general social anxiety. Some artists are inspired by what they see and return home to develop from it; others work while they travel; others make travel their work. The impulse toward constant movement is one more confrontation of that tension, inherent in modern life and in art, between the ephemeral and the permanent—or life and death." —Lucy R. Lippard, Overlay

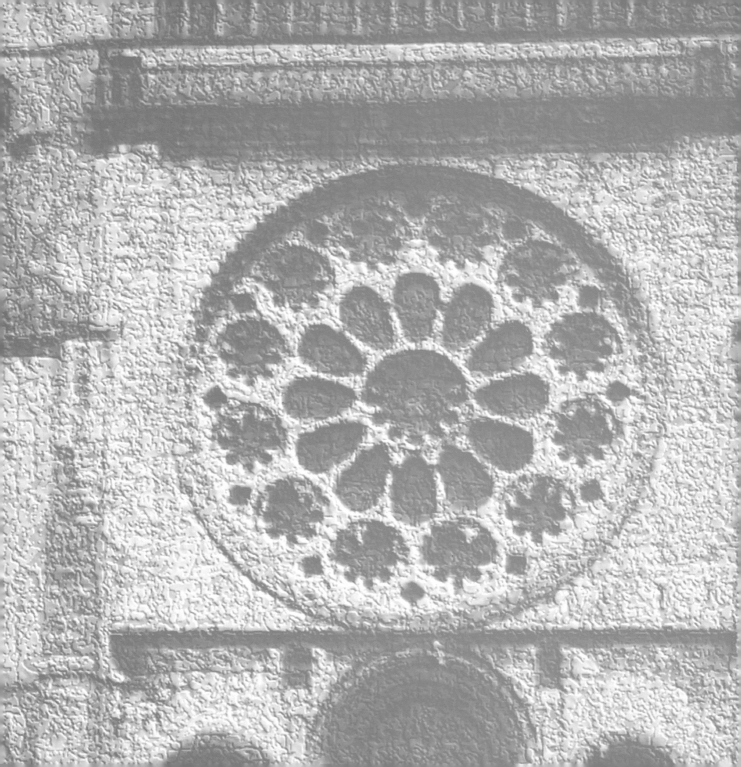

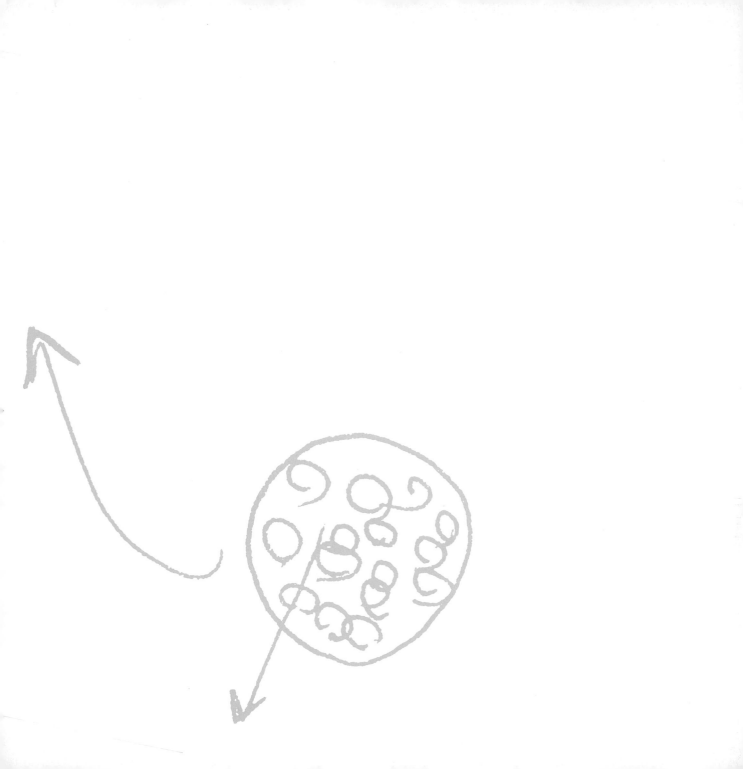

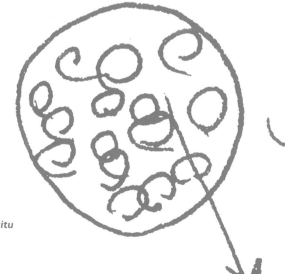

Doctor's drawing of cancer cells *in situ*

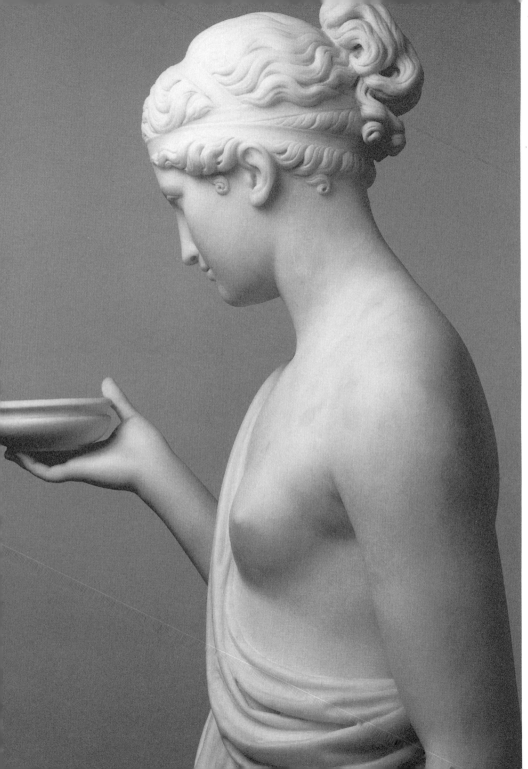

Hebe

Hebe is the cupbearer of the Gods. Without her, the gods would grow old and die. She lives in her far western garden of paradise and governs the Tree of Life, with its magic apples. After the patriarchy and the shift to homosexual romantic love, she is replaced by the youth Ganymede and becomes the constellation Aquarius.

Barbara Walker, *The Woman's Encyclopedia of Myths and Secrets*

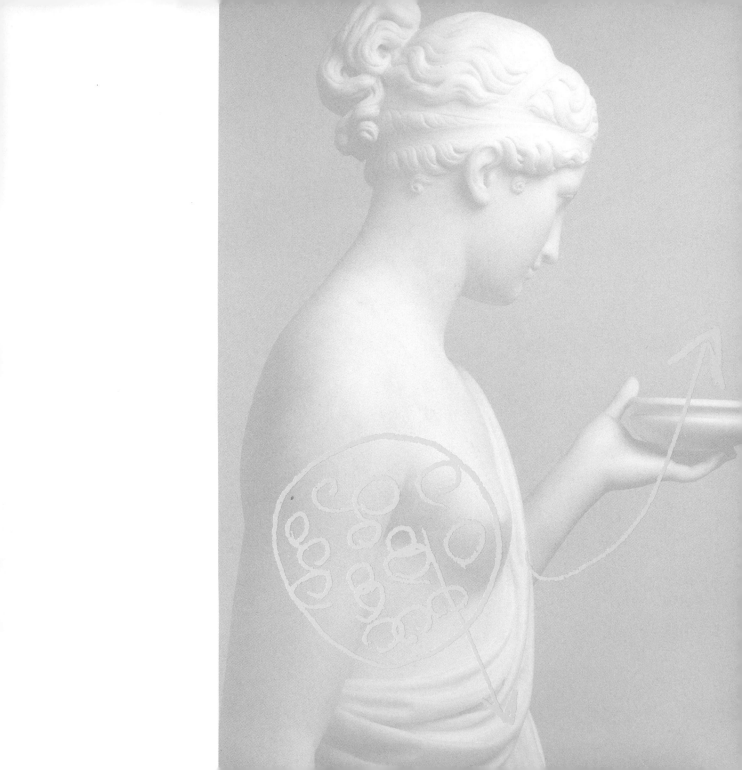

As I head for the door I realize three things: It's already hot at midmorning, it's going to be cooler inside, and if I'm not careful I'll collide with the old man being helped along by the young woman. They are facing me, and although they approach from the opposite direction it's clear we're all headed for the same destination.

It's a split-second decision. I speed up to stay out of their way. It doesn't work. The old man's helper is quick and an expert at pushing the chair. She wheels him around and we are all suddenly there. I unintentionally block their way as we all pause for the electronic eye of the door to acknowledge us, automatically open, and let us enter.

The cool air feels good although it carries the smell of disinfectant. There can be no doubt. I am in it all again. It all begins again. An image in a dream forgotten until it repeats. Although it's been almost three years, all it takes is walking back through these doors. My body remembers these hallways, the experience of this place. Even if I'm acting cool (I feel cooler here), detached, expecting nothing ominous, I start to sweat . . .

Doorway

On this long pilgrimage to remote places, I am still resigned to the impermanence of my human body; if I die on the road it will be the decree of heaven. So thinking, I recovered my vigour a little and stepping out more cheerily passed through the Great Gate of Date.

Basho, *On the Narrow Path to the Deep North*

we are here

I am going on a long trip, far away, and need currency, passport, documents. Special clothes are needed that are both adaptable to unforeseen situations and are presentable. A garment one can sleep in on a train and wear to the opera the next night would be ideal. I make reservations, read a few guidebooks, call my travel agent. How long will it take to go from Amsterdam to Bremen and on to Frankfurt? Should I buy tickets now? I sort everything into clear plastic envelopes, one for each country, one for my art supplies and travel diary. Don't even bother with looking at information on France until ready to go there, almost a month from now. I have a small flat coin purse with three zippers: passport in the deepest, American dollars at the bottom. I won't be needing dollars again until August. I give up known currency. It is only the end of April.

Travel warnings change daily.

After I get sick, I realize there is a strange similarity between being ill and preparing for a long trip. Researching my disease, finding a new doctor, getting second opinions, settling on a course of treatment becomes my full-time job. My life completely changes. I spend most of December and the first part of January in a flurry of appointments to get ready for surgery.

This begins many scenes of waiting, a symphony of waiting. Waiting for news of a phone call down the hall, the first step in finding out whether I have cancer. Waiting for the receptionists to stop cracking jokes and realize I am there.

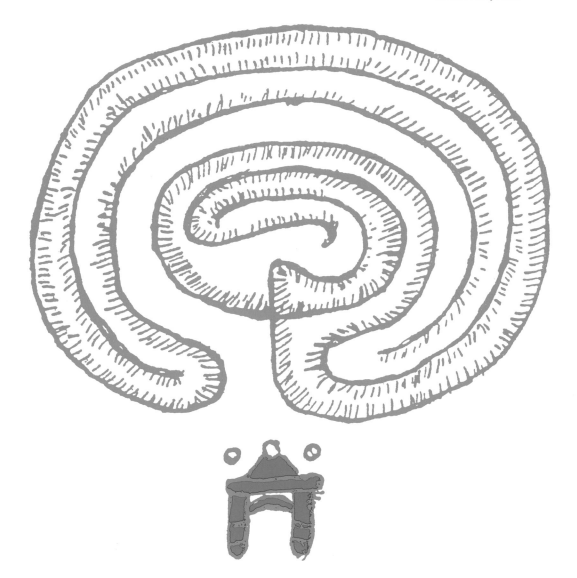

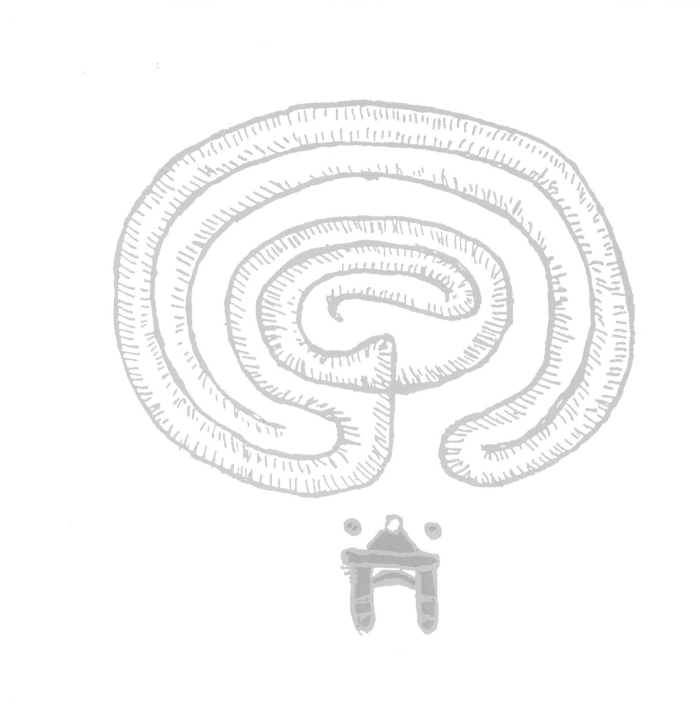

Waiting to schedule a biopsy. Waiting in the outpatient department before 7 A.M., my hands cold from fear and from watering the garden at dawn. Waiting while the staff at the hospital talks about the Christmas party the evening before, as they ready three of us, silent and on gurneys, for surgery. Waiting for news of the biopsy. Waiting over the holiday weekends: The doctor's assistants made a mistake, they won't know anything until Monday. Waiting to hear another opinion on the extent of the cancer. Waiting for the staff in the oncologist's office to make another appointment. Waiting in a room full of people suffering from various stages of cancer, many of whom look sick enough to die. Waiting for surgery. Waiting for someone in the recovery room to pull the blanket up over my knees, I'm not awake enough to remember how to talk or to get their attention. Waiting to hear if they found cancer in my lymph nodes. Waiting for the nurse to find my chart. Waiting to have staples and stitches removed. Waiting for the looks, the responses on people's faces. Waiting until Mike brings round the car. Waiting until Mike has time to help me bathe, to fetch videotapes and groceries from the store. Waiting to be able to drive again. Waiting every day in another dressing room with louvered doors. Waiting to be next in line for radiation therapy. Every day a pink paper gown.

I watch Jaime get ready for her trip, almost a year before I leave. She gives up her apartment and stays with me while we work on a newsletter together. She comes for a week and

Bon Voyage Gifts

On a trip to the local feminist bookstore, I buy her a small labrys for her trip. She leaves me her Schaedler Precision Rules used in her design job and her copy of *The Woman's Encyclopedia of Myths and Secrets.*

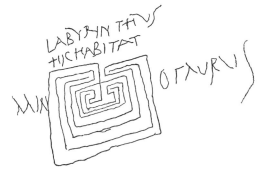

Labrys

n ["an ancient Cretan sacred double ax" — *Webster's*] 1: "The double ax, 'the sign of Imperial might' . . . the symbol of gynocratic power in Crete as it was among the Lycians, the Lydians, the Amazons, the Etruscans, and even the Romans. . . . found in the graves of Paleolithic women of Europe buried 50,000 years ago"

Elizabeth Gould Davis

stays for a month. We delight in reading our twin copies of Mary Daly's *Wickedary*, the intergalactic wicked dictionary, while we sit at my kitchen table and drink tea. She will go and live in Norway, and then travel south to France. I have vague plans. I'm waiting to hear about money to live in France for six months. Her preparations include sorting through books, storing some, shipping some off to Norway where she'll be staying the longest. We both plan to do work on our trips.

At the radiologist's office I am given a booklet. It reminds me of those booklets we got as girls on the changes in our bodies. They had titles like *Growing Up* and were ultimately about menstruation, although there was a subtext. This booklet, subtitled *A Guide to Understanding Breast Problems and Breast Surgery*, shows the girls at middle age and is ultimately about breast cancer. The subtext in this booklet is the number of women who die each year because they don't do breast exams, or have mammograms, or see their doctors (all white men if we believe the pictures here). I skip over the illustrations concerning the stages of a woman's life: a silver-haired matron smiles behind a sheaf of calendar sheets, a middle-aged heterosexual couple enjoy a glass of wine (the man has teeth that are too perfect; he looks like a televangelist), and two women have tea in front of the body of a woman with an undetermined number of breasts. She is undergoing radiation and is faintly rendered, suggesting memory.

The page that scares me is near the end. A disembodied armpit reaches up and reveals a breast that is outlined with a thin black line. This is how much they take for a modified radical mastectomy, this much for a simple mastectomy; "a disadvantage of these operations is that the breast is removed." This much for a partial mastectomy. "The partial mastectomy with axillary dissection removes the tumor and a margin of surrounding healthy tissue. A disadvantage of this procedure includes the necessity of radiation treatment following surgery."

For all the unreality of the other illustrations, these are too real. I am actually scared to turn the page and look at these pictures. It is as if looking at them will mean they will happen, to me. But I do look. I comprehend, through my body, the extent of the various surgeries. These illustrations, packaged in this pamphlet of fluff, help me face what I may have to go through. The rest of it is useless. I go to find a book I bought in England. I stood in the women's bookstore on Charring Cross Road a long time looking at it. Could it only have been last summer? It is an autobiographical account of Jo Spence's life in snapshots and staged photos. Her work is humorous and poignant. I have barely looked at the book since I've come home, but I suddenly remember her photo essay on her own breast cancer. I'd thought her brave to make art out of her illness, yet in the same moment distanced myself from ever having cancer. Surely this would never happen to me.

2: the A-mazing Female Mind that cuts through the double binds and double-binding words of patriarchy; the double ax of Wild wisdom and wit that breaks through the mazes of man-made mystification, cutting the mindbindings of master-minded doublethink; Power of Discernment which divines the difference between Reality and unreality, between the Natural Wild and elemental fabrications.

Mary Daly

Amazon Lore

It is thought that Amazons burned off their right breasts so they had increased flexibility in their arm and were better able to use the bow and arrow. Their weapons included the labrys, or double ax, a shield in the shape of the half moon, the spear and the bow. The double ax was a symbol of the Great Mother, the double ax between the moon-shaped horns of the sacred bull.

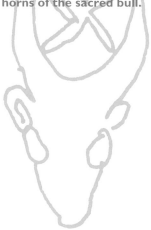

I had to go into hospital. Suddenly. Dutifully, so as not to waste time, I took with me several books on theories of representation, a thin volume on health and a historical novel. One morning, while reading, I was confronted by the awesome reality of a young white-coated doctor, with student retinue, standing by my bedside. As he referred to his notes, without introduction, he bent over me and began to ink a cross onto the area of flesh above my left breast. As he did so a whole chaotic series of images flashed through my head. Rather like drowning. I heard this doctor, whom I had never met before, this potential daylight mugger, tell me that my left breast would have to be removed. Equally I heard myself answer, 'No'. Incredulously; rebelliously; suddenly; angrily; attackingly; pathetically; alone; in total ignorance. I who had spent three years (and more) immersed in a study of ideology and visual representation, now suddenly needed another type of knowledge. . . . Jo Spence.

Susan's husband has died and I've suffered losses as well since we traveled together in England a few years ago. The breeziness of Holland is a change from the arid climates of Cairo and California. She is still in mourning. I need to step out of my normal life and take this journey. I need time alone, away from the demands of others and my life in L.A. I'm glad to see Susan again but also glad that I don't, after another week, have to travel with anyone else until late June. I've given myself three months in Europe, England and Ireland, a shortened sabbatical. Maybe it is working. I already start to feel calm.

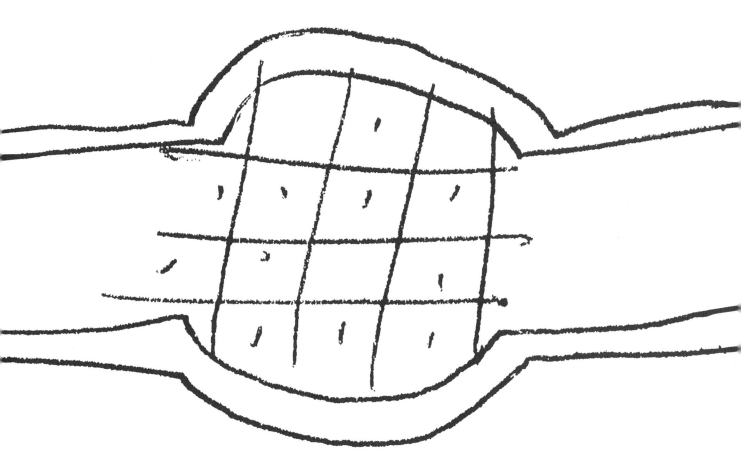

Doctor's drawing of cancer
expanding in duct.

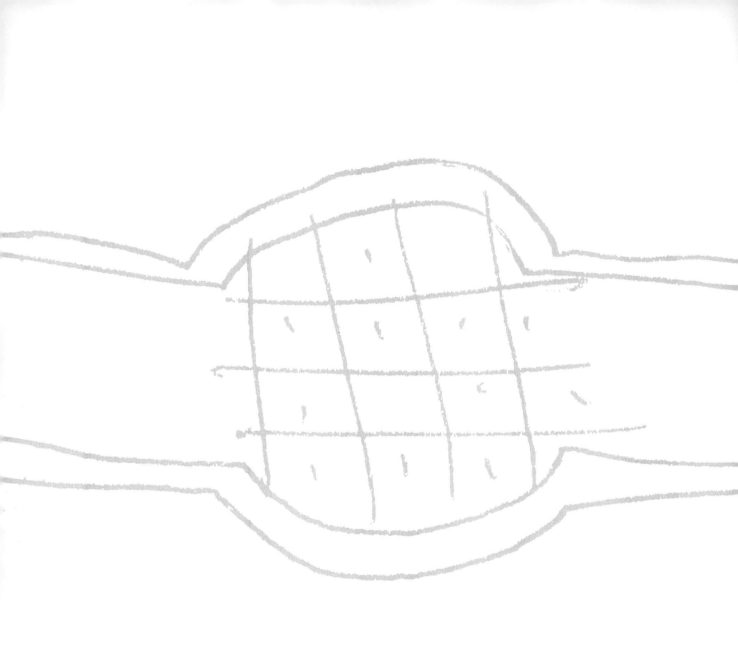

In April I flew to Holland + traveled by train to Bremen. Drove on to Worpswede. Then Frankfurt + Mainz for bookshow. All of May in Paris.

I hooked up with Calligraphy tour in London to look at medieval Manuscripts in England and Ireland. Spent a week looking at The Book of Kells + going to sites such as Tara + New Grange. Drove through Wales w/ Allwynn, Carmel + Kathleen. We drove on the other side of the road and looked at Standing Stones.

Now I am involved in a different journey. It is more disorienting than driving on the wrong side of The road.

Fly from California to London to Amsterdam. Start in Holland. Sleep away a whole afternoon and evening. Meet Susan the next morning for breakfast at the small hotel in an old canal house. She is just back from Egypt, ending her trip as I begin mine. We eat in a large room that overlooks the small garden.

We step out of our small hotel and go no farther than the next doorway. The windows of the basement storefront sparkle. The pristine shop is filled with antique samplers from America and Europe. Susan forges ahead, and I find myself in the shop, surrounded by samplers of various sizes. Another customer sits at a table, magnifying glass in hand, counting threads or stitches on a sampler in a thin gold frame. Susan and I are both drawn to the unusual ones that have large cross shapes sewn onto linen. Mr. Coenders, the owner, tells us these are darning samplers. Darning samplers are made by slitting the cloth. The goal is to create a decorative but invisible repair, done by approximating weaving patterns. Some are small, abstract designs done in colored thread recreating plaids. Some crosses are white on white and practically invisible.

My money has been carefully parceled out for the next three months. But I know I will buy one of the darning samplers. I know this feeling from shopping flea markets, know I should pay attention to it. Some purchases are momentous. And I've found a memento for my entire trip on the first morning. The darning sampler I like has a scattered design, not the usual tightly organized pattern seen on most samplers. It has more spirit because of its randomness. I will economize some other way.

I spend many days in May looking at needlework. On this trip, tapestries and embroideries hold more fascination for me than painting. On one of my first days in Paris I visit Gobelins

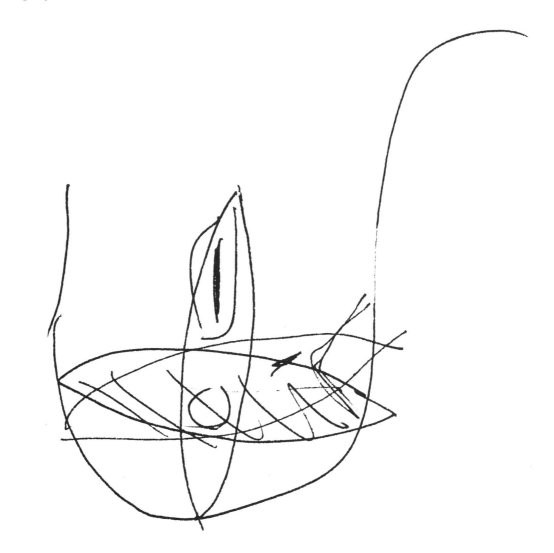

Surgeon's drawing of possible incisions.

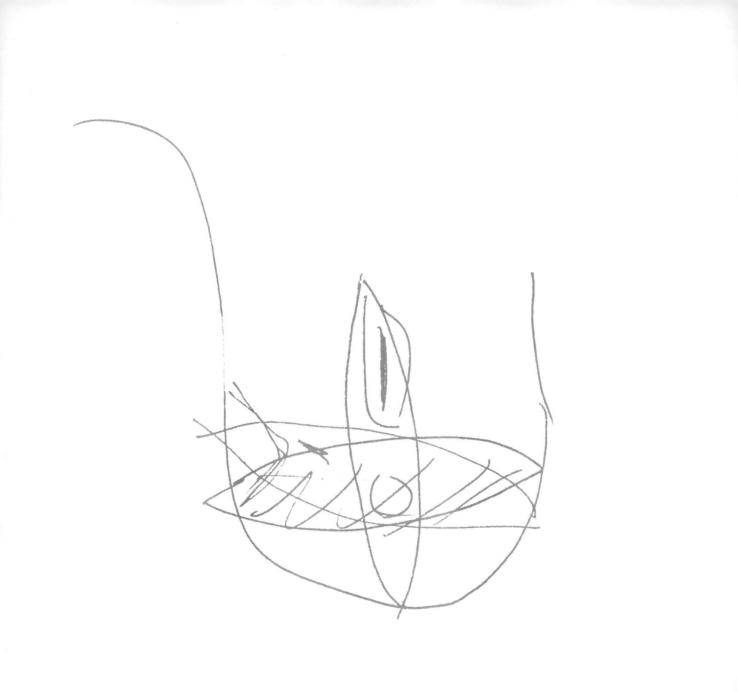

workshops, the famous tapestry studio where tapestry is still being made in the traditional manner. I write Shelley a postcard, describing the giant wood looms that remind me of the sewing frames used in bookbinding. Here they have grown huge. June and July, in England and Ireland, I spend looking at ancient books, laced together with vellum strips, all decorated by hand. A week at Trinity College in Dublin is spent looking at *The Book of Kells* and drawing the swirls of this and other Celtic manuscripts.

At the plastic surgeon's office in early December, I am struck by the decor. On my first few visits, I think of it as a kind of nightclub. Low tables, comfortable couches, flower arrangements, and flattering lighting. I have been in such clinical surroundings since the biopsy that I'm taken aback at this plush waiting room. My first visit here is to explore options in case I have a mastectomy. Since my life has been taken over by medical appointments, one more won't matter. My oncologist has sent me to this particular doctor. The oncologist is the first person I have felt comfortable with, although her news isn't all that good. She thinks I might have cancer that has spread. She is still looking at and interpreting information, and I am here on her recommendation. As I really look at the chairs and rugs, the art on the wall, I realize that everything here is woven, stitched up. Not the refinement of European tapestry but the gutsy textiles of the Americas. Fragments of a Pre-Columbian weaving hang on the wall.

International Call

My father figures out the phone system well enough to call me from Kentucky to tell me my mother has just had a biopsy and that she has breast cancer. They have removed her breast, and she is doing well. I am in shock from this news.

If the girl making the darning sampler did a bad job, her teacher made the slit, the area of repair, bigger.

Repressions and Rebellion

In that torn bit of brown leather brace worked through and through with yellow silk, in that bit of white rag with the invisible stitching lying among fallen leaves and rubbish that the wind has blown into the gutter or street corner, lies all the passing of some woman's soul finding voiceless expression. Has the pen or pencil dipped so deep in the blood of the human race as the needle?

Olive Shreiner quote, samplers exhibit, Oxfordshire, June 1989

A woven and stitched rustic rug is underfoot. It's not museum quality, but a fitting choice for a group of nimble-fingered plastic surgeons.

The plastic surgeon is from Texas. She is very present and looks directly at me as I tell her my story to this point. I find it extraordinary to be sitting in the giant orange insect-like lounge chair of the examining room. I have trouble staying in my body. I am still in such shock from this whole ordeal. I can barely believe I am talking to her about cutting my breast again—I have a mastectomy yet to undure. The choices for breast reconstruction are a silicone implant and a procedure called the tram flap, where tissue is moved from my stomach to create a new breast of my living tissue. If I don't undergo a total mastectomy, one possibility is a reduction of my other breast, to give me two breasts that are similar in size. She asks some questions I can't answer: Will I have a nipple left? She can create one. I return to the waiting room, the room of textile fragments, where I wait with a few still very beautiful older women, here, obviously, for face-lifts. I had planned to grow old like the painter Alice Neel or the photographer Imogen Cunningham, with a face full of wrinkles, with my breasts intact. I had planned to grow old.

I've lost spoken English by the third week in Paris. I am out of practice. On many days I speak to no one except vendors selling fruit and vegetables on rue Rambuteau or to ticket sellers at the museum or film I'll go to that day. Then it is usually in French. *Un billet, je dit.* I cup my hands to indicate

My drawing of stitches on rug in waiting room.

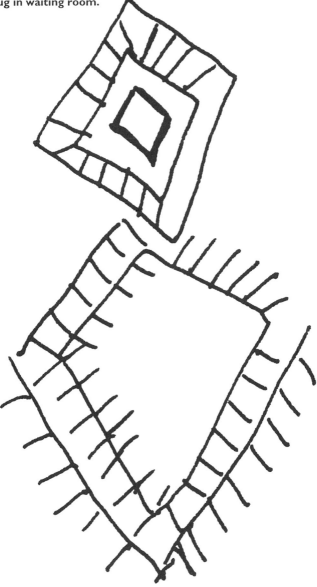

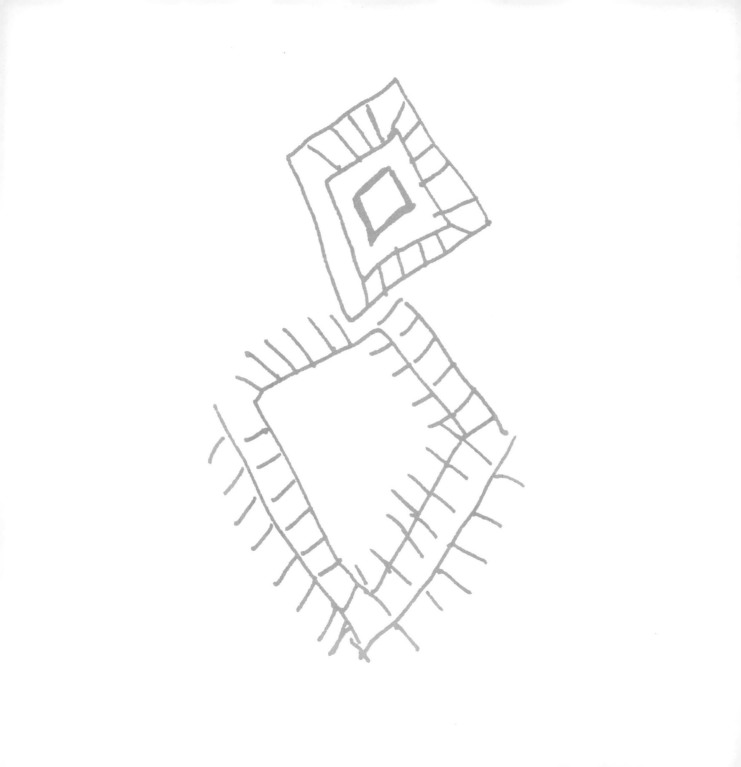

how many cherries. *Je dit, Un comme ça.* I point at stalks of pale, fat asparagus wrapped in twine, a bunch of grapes, a carton of raspberries. I nod and say *Bonjour* when I see my neighbors: two young construction workers gutting the artists' apartment in the adjoining building, and an older woman with a witless little dog on a leash. They are often standing in the courtyard when I go out. I usually stop and pet the little dog. I talk to the dog in English.

It is not so much speaking my own language I miss, as understanding what is going on around me. I sit in cafés and miss whole conversations at the next table. I catch words, phrases, but sentences are simply spoken too fast. I sit and watch. I watch couples enjoying meals, friends talking over café express, women nodding and smiling as men talk on and on. I see tourists, like myself, in various states of bafflement or enjoyment in the café adjacent to a museum or in a nearby *salon de thè* (tea salon). Language is critical when it comes to ordering food or understanding the life of the street.

I go to the movies to hear English. The French, purist film buffs that they are, show most movies in v.o., *version originale.* Many of the three hundred movies shown each week in Paris are excellent prints in the original language. Subtitles are in French. On the last trip, even this proved difficult. Whole German sections of *Sophie's Choice* were translated into French subtitles. In *Mishima*, I scrambled to translate French subtitles while listening to Japanese. It's been raining for the last few days. I go to see *Rain Man.*

Voix Originale

— And why do you go to France and Belgium, said Miss Ivors, instead of visiting your own land?

— Well, said Gabriel, it's partly to keep in touch with the languages and partly for a change.

— And haven't you your own language to keep in touch with — Irish? asked Miss Ivors.

— Well, said Gabriel, if it comes to that, you know, Irish is not my language.

James Joyce, *The Dead*

Mostly I go to the movies at night, after the museums and shops close. But since Paris has turned cold and wet, I've taken refuge in the movies. Three people at the matinee of *La Route des Indes* (*Passage to India*). I am catching up on years of missed movies. On a rainy Friday night I decide to venture far afield to an early show at a revival theater on the lower edge of Montparnasse. Before I leave the neighborhood, I go to a Chinese restaurant recommended by the artists next door. I've been there once. But today, because it's early, I stumble into the restaurant out of the rain to find myself the only customer there to eat a bowl of soup. The restaurant is occupied by a group of Chinese men, all chain-smoking and drinking strong tea, all intrigued by the never-ending series of stories by the main storyteller, in full control of his audience. To them, I don't exist. I can't understand a word. I sip my soup and look out on the early rainy evening in this alleyway of Paris.

The theater in Montparnasse is tiny. Stepping up to buy a ticket in the minuscule lobby I notice a giant take-up reel, for the movie now showing, revolving over the head of the ticket seller. The projection booth must be tinier still. The schedule is a jumble, as far as I can tell; there are two theaters showing a list of ever-changing movies. It reminds me of a theater my youngest brother might run. He spends all his creativity on ideas, little on his surroundings. He would love this bleak place and its ever-changing roster of movies. It is raining, and although a few of us who are early stand in the

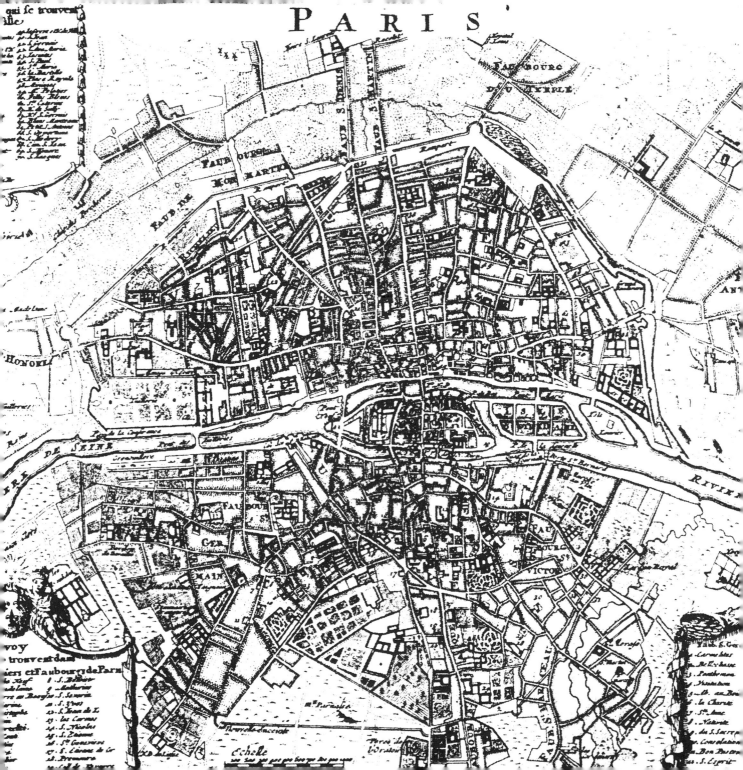

PARIS

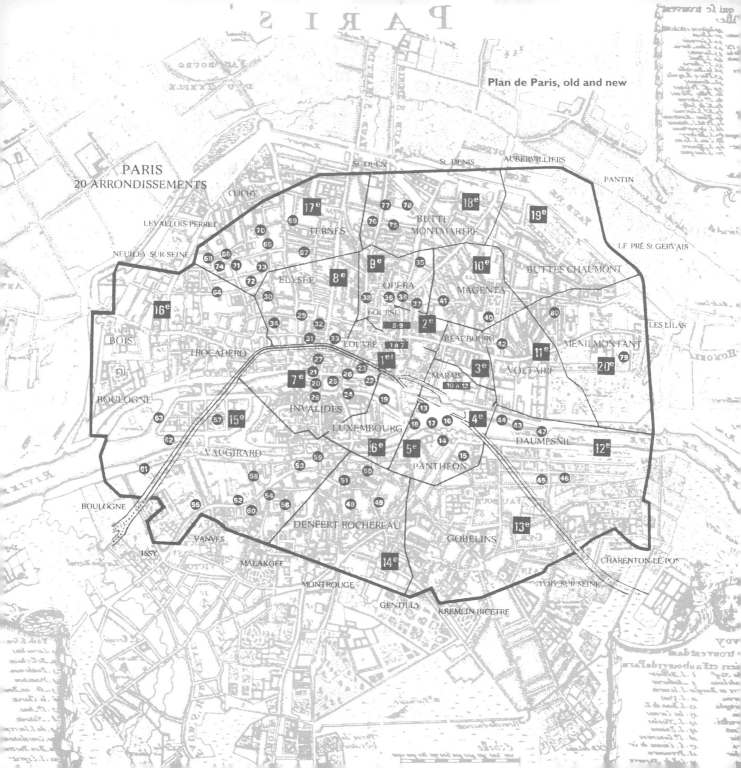

PARIS

Plan de Paris, old and new

PARIS
20 ARRONDISSEMENTS

shelter of the lobby, we are eventually shooed back into the rain by a torrent of abuse from the ticket seller. The tiny lobby remains empty while we stand, most of us bareheaded, in the rain. Finally in the cave-like theater, we sit and look at a screen to our left.

This theater, where one has the feeling of sitting in a hole, is occupied by patrons who are conspicuous and identifiable as English speaking, although most of them aren't talking. English has brought us to this place, a subterranean haven, where, for two hours, we are lost and absorbed in *Les Gens de Dublin* (*The People of Dublin*, a translation of Joyce's collection of short stories entitled *Dubliners*, which contains the story *The Dead*, the basis for this movie.). The words flood over me. I am overwhelmed by the beauty of his writing, by the characters, by the spoken language, after a month of English as a second language. I have chosen this movie because I will be in Dublin in a month. It proves to be more than just background material for the next part of my trip. In these two hours I've understood something fundamental about my father's Irish family. I know these aunts, renowned for their hospitality, from some deep place. My father's foster mother could have been one of these women, had her family stayed in Ireland, had they not come to America and grown tall. And, in a strange way, I've recognized something about Joyce, publishing *Dubliners* when he was in self-imposed exile in Paris. How much closer he must have felt to the beauty of Ireland. One turns back to see what one has had to leave, and its beauty shines brighter.

Chinese Restaurant

Christmas Day, and neither of us have planned anything beyond opening gifts. We have been busy with my medical crisis. We usually visit Mike's family, but not this year. We go to the movies. Most of the Jewish community seems to be there this morning. We end up at one of the few local restaurants open, a Chinese restaurant down the street. The place is almost empty. Our young waiter is new at this. He's as awkward as we are.

Hometown Movies

After I get better, I go to see *The Doctor,* a movie about a surgeon who gets cancer. There is the usual Hollywood take on life: The young woman who becomes his friend is too beautiful and too wise. We all know she will die before the movie is over. One part they get right. He is in a crowded elevator. Everyone rushes off at the first floor, getting on with their busy lives. The doors close. He goes, alone, to the radiation clinic in the basement.

Not quite in Hollywood. I have been here before. There is too much pink and wicker. The decor is a cross between a bed and breakfast of the 1980s with watered-down Laura Ashley furnishings, and a ladies' powder room in a better department store circa 1950. But there is something fundamentally askew. The sweet powdery smell is there to mask the smell of chemicals, of a darkroom on the other side of the wall. And a darkened room with lightboxes on the wall for viewing mammograms sits off the interior hallway. I am let into the changing room of pastel, louvered doors and plush carpeting. The gown has been washed so many times, it takes me three tries to decide which side should face out. I feel vulnerable and I cling to this shred of self-composure: not wearing the gown wrong side out in public. In this case, out into the public space of the hallway. I wait my turn for a routine mammogram, a bit impatient because tomorrow is Thanksgiving and I am anxious to be done with errands. It doesn't dawn on me, when they call me back, twice, for more films, that anything is wrong. I accept the technician's lie that I have moved, breathed in with the heavy machine bearing down, squeezing my breasts, when I shouldn't have breathed at all. After I've read an insipid magazine from cover to cover, they tell me that the radiologist wants to see me. They've found something suspicious. I finally do it right; I stop breathing.

He points to this map of my breast. The calcifications, enlarged, look like specks of dandruff. I appreciate his showing me the films, his careful explanation, tempered with grave concern, that I follow this up, that I follow the films up, that I do something immediately. He wants to see other films right away. It becomes clear that it will be quicker for me to call the two doctors I've seen and collect the films, my films, from their archives. I am my own gopher, here, south of Hollywood.

Mid-December. I find a small paper garland in the week between undergoing my biopsy and hearing the results. It depicts the Virgin Mary and the Annunciation angel, Gabriel. The garland is made in Germany and is a series of arched panels that open, accordion-like; the same painting in miniature is printed over and over, to achieve a festive Christmas effect. It catches my eye because the angel is so small, no bigger than a flying squirrel, hovering midair, to the left of the Virgin. I realize, with increasing horror, that I too wait for the annunciation. The annunciation by my doctor, this very day. With this realization, the small paper decoration takes on tremendous power. I quickly put it back on the shelf. I don't want today's appointment to be so symbolic. I don't want to find omens here at the hardware store. And since I have, I won't buy it.

What is left out of the Annunciation scene? Surely Gabriel had a helper, an angel, his best friend, a secretary or nurse standing out in the hall, outside the frame. Someone to make and break appointments, set the stage, make sure Mary was seated when she heard the news that her life was to be trans-

The Annunciation

From this moment on, I alternate between the moods, passive and accepting, scared, and angry and wild. The next three weeks are chaotic: Make appointments, make phone calls, read about cancer, break some appointments and make others. Can I be seen right away? But we are stuck in a frozen picture plane: Nothing is decided. Only at night I panic. I wake up screaming from a nightmare that someone is breaking into our house. A few nights later, my husband has the same dream.

formed. I didn't need to be seated to hear what the doctor had to say. The nurse's face said it all. I had cancer. I knew I would have to endure the look on her face many times over on other faces. It scared and angered me almost more than having cancer. I didn't wanted to be treated with pity.

The interview with the doctor was cool. There were cancer cells up to the edge of the biopsy. He wasn't sure he'd cut out all the cancer. His cure: cut my breast off, perhaps both breasts as a preventative measure. He added the second breast almost as an afterthought, as if he were talking about hangnails or some benign procedure. Like Mary, I was stunned when I heard the news. There were signs I probably had cancer—I fit the profile well. Deep in thought, I remember staring intently at his hands, and his ballpoint pen as he sat at his fancy desk. He talked nonstop and scribbled nervously on a notepad. An old friend, now dead of AIDS, used to look at my pensive face, laugh and say, "And Mary pondered these things in her heart."

It always made me furious when he said that. This doctor makes me furious. I am angry he didn't do a better job. I had dye injected into my breast to show him where to cut. He is so nonchalant in suggesting I cut off my breasts. It is obvious I can't trust him. Women's intuition. I knew this from my first visit there, when he stood at the sink in the examining room with his back to me and took my medical history. Why didn't I listen to myself instead of the others who give him glowing reports as a surgeon? And listen I did. I pondered my

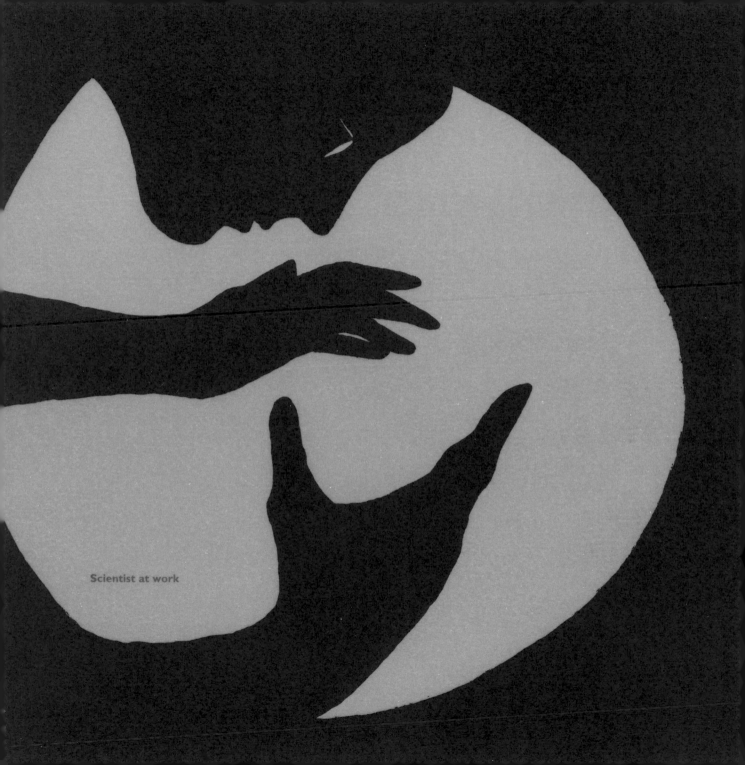

Scientist at work

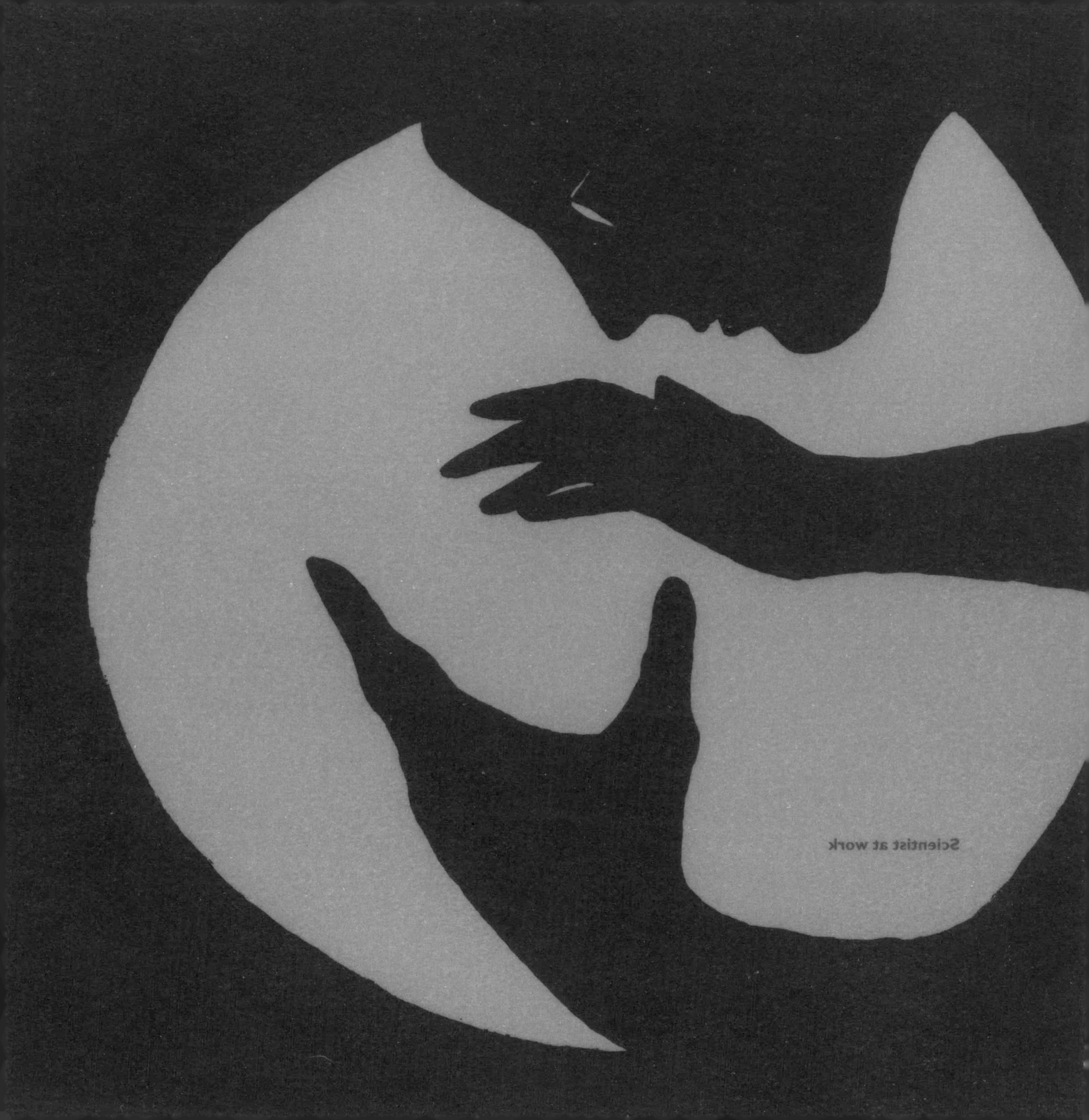

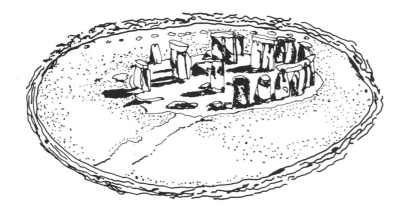

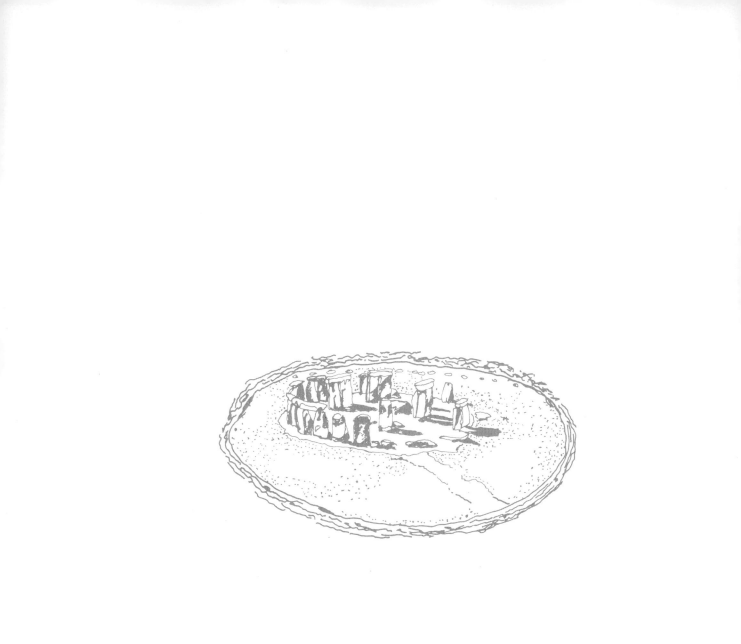

motives for not trusting him, and quieted the anxiety I felt about him, about this whole situation. I am angry that we live in a world where women's breasts are cut and discarded in this casual way. I need to know the extent of this treatment. And so it begins. Mary sits in a frozen scene. Her life, my life, will forever be divided into two halves, before and after this moment. Mary, in this incarnation as the future mother of God, is picture perfect and passive. I maintain this pose until I hit the sidewalk outside the medical center. It has turned dark and cold, as if, here on this ordinary night in December, someone has turned out the light and heat of the entire world.

When I look for the paper garland later, weeks later, like all omens ignored, it is gone.

Thursday, Winter Solstice, I am in another doctor's examining room overlooking a street I've driven down many times. I see the city planner's intent from this overview. It takes on a completely different feeling from this height. I'd never imagined this car-clogged street as the palm-lined boulevard it clearly is. It stretches toward the ocean. This is the most dramatic view so far. All this week has been spent in doctors' offices. The views from the examining room windows have given me new appreciation for this sprawling city of shifting light on stucco walls. Palm trees in winter. Our family never wintered in Florida, but there are photos of my handsome grandfather there, on some beach, with my dad's extended family. This year it looks like I will be wintering in the land of

Ancient and medieval labyrinths or mazes . . . presume a double perspective: maze-treaders, whose vision ahead and behind is severely constricted and fragmented, suffer confusion, whereas maze-viewers who see the pattern whole, from above or in a diagram, are dazzled by its complex artistry.

cancer. The first part of this pilgrimage is to visit as many medical sites throughout the city as possible.

Today is Winter Solstice. The shortest day of the year. Here, even though the window faces east, I know the sun is about to set over the Pacific. The last patient of the day, here at the end of the pagan year, I wait to see another surgeon. Resigned more than hopeful, I look down. I am wearing yet another cloth gown. Many pilgrims walked the pilgrim's road barefoot, as penance for their sins. Only people convicted of serious crimes walked the pilgrim's route in sack cloth and ashes. The pilgrims felt a need to announce their purpose as strangers in foreign territories. When one undertakes a journey this large, there should be special clothing to mark it from ordinary life. These cloth and paper hospital gowns are my winter wardrobe, my pilgrim's garb. At times, I feel all I need do is take off the gown, put on my street clothes, and walk out.

I don't expect much from this visit. It is Thursday. I always feel somehow protected or cushioned by week's end, now more than ever. I've made it through another week without surgery. After this appointment, I'm meeting my niece, an artist. We have a date to see a movie at the museum. I don't know it yet, but by the time I meet her in an hour things will have changed. I know from the minute I meet this doctor that he is a healer. His treatment plan is much less radical. He actually says I don't have to lose my breast unless he discovers more cancer. He seems to have some idea what that means,

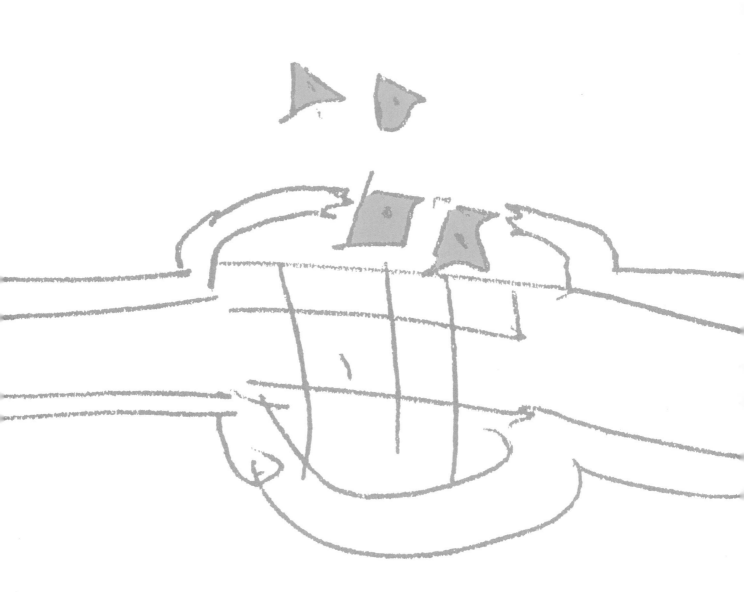

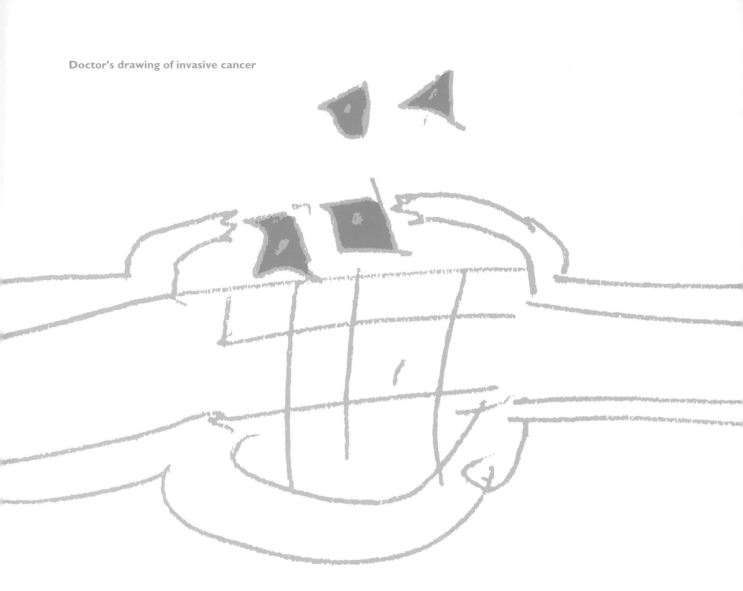

Doctor's drawing of invasive cancer

losing one's breast. He spends a long time talking to me and carefully looks over everything I've brought. He wants more information. Retrieving pathology slides and reports from the hospital across town is my assignment for the Friday before the holiday week. He is Jewish. I look at him skeptically when he tells me to go home and try to have a nice Christmas holiday. We both know there is no vacation from this, but from this moment, from sunset on, I feel as if I am in ritual time.

The wind whips across the asphalt at the Farmer's Market. All the stalls and shops are closing. Huge, perfect oranges and mounds of dates are covered up for the night. We sit at the lunch counter of a trendy café and eat our quick dinner that has been hastily cooked. I am so glad to see Rachel, to be doing something ordinary. I always forget she is almost young enough to be my daughter. She is wise beyond her years. The food is good, if a bit underdone. It is freezing, and we snuggle closer. We laugh at the food, and at the absurdity of dining al fresco on the first night of winter. Once inside the theater, she pulls out a small package. She and her new husband have bought me a tiny silver angel. I must wear it over my ailing breast, she says, a guardian angel, to protect me during my surgery and treatment.

Neither of us know it yet, but Rachel becomes a kind of guardian angel. I can't yet step back from the Annunciation painting to know she is the one standing just outside the picture plane. In the coming months, she misses school, takes a day off work, drives her art truck to Los Angeles to make

What you see depends on where you stand, and thus, at one and the same time, labyrinths are single (there is one physical structure) and double: they simultaneously incorporate order and disorder, clarity and confusion, unity and multiplicity, artistry and chaos.

Penelope Reed Doob

The Palm Tree

In the Babylonian myth of
the primal garden, the palm
tree was the Tree of Life, a
dwelling-place of the
Goddess Astarte. The
Hebrew version of her
name was Tamar, "Palm
Tree."

*The Woman's Encyclopedia of Myths
and Secrets*

Pilgrims in the Middle Ages,
on their way home from
Palestine, stuck a palm
frond in their hats and were
known as "palmers."

cornmeal and blueberry muffins with me. She arrives in thrift store dresses and boots and is even more radical in her assessment of the doctors than I am. We watch videotapes of obscure movies sent by my brother in Florida. I sleep, and she watches over me.

Friends circle around. People I haven't talked to in years call or write to say they've been thinking a lot about me lately. Is everything OK? The news is carried on the ether. Some pass over the awkward part of the conversation by telling me about their friend, the famous writer or celebrated archeologist, who has had cancer. They never really ask me how I am. A few never call. Michael, my husband, knows too much because of his medical training. He misreads one report and, for a week, is sure I will die. When he realizes my prognosis is excellent, he relaxes. He wants everything returned to normal, our normal life back. He is hopeful about my recovery but doesn't comprehend the trauma my body and psyche are going through. Medical school didn't teach him that. I become adept at taking care of myself.

One day after Winter Solstice. The tinted colors of the glass slides beam when held up under fluorescent lights, a poor substitute for noonday sun in this critical time of the year. The shapes on the slides are amorphous, with the surprise of the organic built into their irregularities. I now hold in my hand striking color combinations, small flakes of matter and odd bits of microscopic pieces I will never know the names of, but can see, can be amazed by.

Labyrinth at Chartres

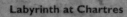
Labyrinth at Chartres

The effect is achieved by staining and dyeing human tissue, my tissue. The tissue, the wait for the results, the frightening consequences of this horrifying journey have become for this moment only small surrealist jewels, wrapped in a box for me to take home, three days before Christmas.

The pathology lab is feebly decorated for the holidays. The pristine counters, the snow-white ambiance of the corridors speak to artificially created environments, those of unsettling dreams more than festive occasions. The few remaining workers who haven't finagled this Friday off are frazzled and distracted, in limbo. Uncaring conductors on the French train system forced to work holidays. Because this time doesn't really count, they seem resentful of having to be here.

I have to be here.

All through this holiday season I've encountered droves of holiday shoppers and have been as busy as any of them. But instead of shopping for Christmas Eve dinner and small presents to fill stockings, I have been shopping for cures, for surgeons, for bits of medical information, for my own X-rays lost by the hospital or the doctor (they blame one another), for cancer specialists, for peace of mind/piece of mind.

The slides look like stained glass.

That Thursday in Paris it suddenly turned hot, so that on the way from the Musée d'Orsay back to rue des Archives I stop in a big department store near the Seine to buy a hat. I suddenly decide to leave town the next day and go to Chartres. Buying the hat is a marker of my emotional state, a

In Transit

My new best friend is the parking lot attendant. We get the same days off from the clinic: weekends & holidays, and we always have something to say to one another about the weather or traffic.

The Wheel of Fortune

Northern Europeans believed the mystic wheels of existence stopped turning at the crucial transition from one year to the next, during the darkest days of winter, when the sun came to its nadir. At this time, during the season of Yule, all rotating motions were taboo.

The Woman's Encyclopedia of Myths and Secrets

different attitude I've come to that morning. The group singing for money in the Metro car put me in a good mood for the rest of the day. I realize I better enjoy as much of the trip as I can. After a month away, I feel settled into this experience. Whatever has been clinging to me, holding me back, on my back, is gone. Winter is gone. The hat is for all the sunny days ahead.

Getting to the train the next morning was a descent through purgatory. The Montparnasse train station was being wrenched apart by dozens of workmen deconstructing the city. Dust from defeated concrete was everywhere and the noise was deafening, but there was nowhere to go but on. At the edge of reconstruction, I found a makeshift ticket window and asked, in French, for a ticket and return to Chartres. The ticket agent looks quizzical. I'm not sure if it is my French or my new French hat that provoked his startled look. I notice with dismay that I am beginning to catalog the body language and facial expressions of total strangers, perhaps because I depend on their kindness.

Finding out where it is on the map, climbing the stairs or locating the elevator after getting there, figuring out how to get there so I'll be there on time, or at least not too late. Showing my card, my ticket, or paying admission, filling out some form or some combination of all four. Figuring out the money.

I finally locate the right track. The train is almost empty and hot. It will be a while before we reach Chartres. We lurch

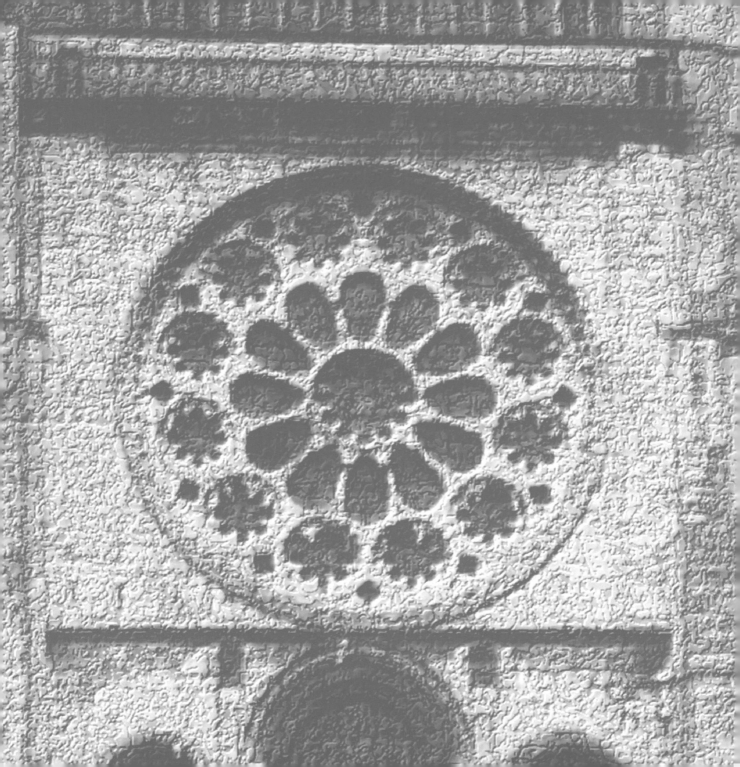

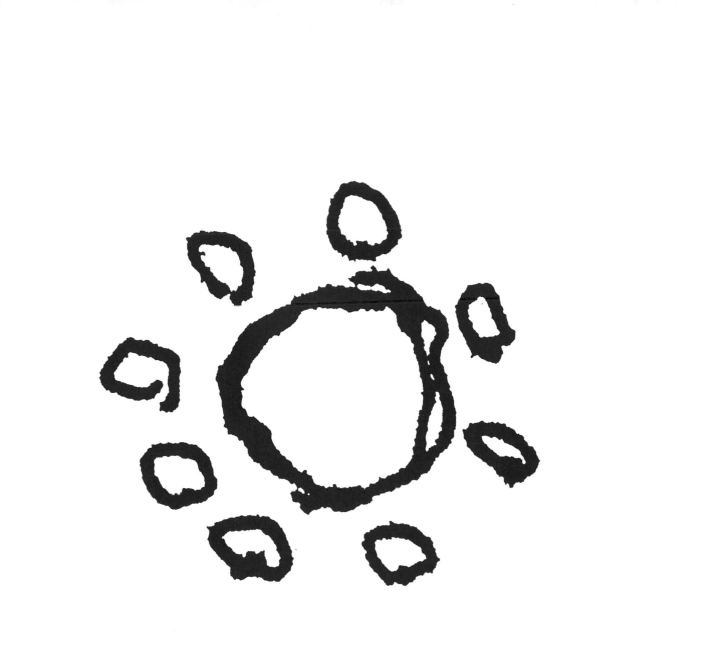

My drawing, radiation on wall, radiation room

forward. The pilgrims, on their way on an ordinary day to see the great rose windows of the greatest cathedral in France, include a French couple, a blind man by himself, a family speaking German and suffering from the heat, and me.

Our first view of Chartres is from the windows of the train. When Mike and I saw Stonehenge across Salisbury Plain we were awestruck. I've forgotten about the tremendous body rush at seeing these monuments from the moment they appear on the horizon. It is always a surprise. In minutes we are on the hot sidewalk in front of the train station. Most paths lead up to the cathedral. The sun glares and beats down on the stones in front of the church. But with the first step inside Chartres, I am plunged into a dark, deep reality, as if I'd been sucked in, pulled, from the bright white light of the plaza, into the deep cool interior. Here one is truly inside looking out. Our guide, Malcolm Miller, a permanent fixture of the Cathedral for years, talks of the cathedral as a book, with the sculpture and windows as its text. As he talks, most of the English-speaking tourists look up at the magnificent stained glass windows. While they look up, I look down to the great labyrinth on the stone floor. It is partially covered with chairs. It is placed below the western rose window that portrays the Last Judgment. Pilgrims to Chartres, who couldn't make the trip on to Jerusalem, followed the path of this labyrinth on their knees. The rose shape at the center of the labyrinth echoes the rose window above it. Some believe there was originally a metal plate at

A Deep Reality

I am quickly in a deep meditation because of acupressure. She says, *Imagine a circle of light drawn around the hospital, the bed, the surgical instruments.* Barbara has been both practitioner and teacher to me. I realized I would go on sabbatical to Europe this year during one of her treatments. Now we are embarked on a different but similar journey. And, as with the awe of visiting New Grange and Chartres, there are no words.

Archetypally, to untangle something is to make a descent, to follow a labyrinth, to descend into the underworld or the place where things are revealed in an entirely new way, to be able to follow a convoluted process.

Clarissa Pinkola Estés

———

the center on which there was an image of the Minotaur, linking it to the labyrinth at Crete.

My name is checked at the counter, and I am routed down the hall to room three. The halls are long and endless from this perspective—dreamlike. I will never find my way back through this maze. Although there is no large crowd, I am being pushed forward. There is the sensation of not being able to turn around and go back. Plus I am tangled up in all this equipment, and someone's taken my shoes. I look down at my body. My street clothes are gone as well. Flat on my back on the gurney, my landmarks are variations in the patterns on the ceiling. The ceiling becomes an upside down path, speeding by.

As my course of radiation begins, I am lead, every morning, down the ramp to the tomb underground. The workers take my paper smock and arrange my breast and neck to align with the red lasers. The blue drawings on my body must line up perfectly with the red lines that ricochet around the room. I am partially clothed in the lead apron. My head must remain still and in a fixed position, looking up to heaven, the posture of devotion. They leave, closing the heavy door behind them. I am alone. Looking up, high on the wall, I can see the small rosettes of the lasers. The noise of the radiation starts. At first it is a high buzzing sound, then the noise changes to low chanting sound. I spend my moments inside the sealed chamber counting the petals of the rosettes, about all I can see with my head at this angle. I suddenly know the lasers are connected by some universal law of design to the great rose windows at Chartres.

I am on the verge of being sickened or reassured by the pattern on the chairs in the waiting room. I am already dazed from the flu, from waiting for this appointment, from no lunch, from sitting in this room on chairs that have radiation waves permanently woven into their tapestry skin. Some designer's scheme or a joke? Surely this cannot be meant: a radiologist's office decorated in complementary colors that dance before the eyes of irradiated patients. Even the business cards are printed in these vibrating colors.

The doctor is running late. After an hour I am finally admitted into his inner office, one of several offices that ring a circular desk, a central command post lifted from the set of outer space movies, meant to suggest the latest in technology, efficiency and control in the exploration of unknown territory. His office opens off central command and is black, chrome, wood. Shells sit on glass shelves. Nature in a pristine, ordered form. A chambered nautilus cut in half. His job: seeing inside.

We learn to draw trees from an art teacher who comes only once to our fifth-grade class. On this special day, we are allowed out before recess to sit at the foot of the oak tree and learn the proper formula. The tree we are to draw is in a forbidden part of the school yard, near the portico of white columns and the stunted circular drive that links the school

Radiation Tapestry

The plum and green of early spring, the colors of China, and Eloise Klein Healy's book of poetry based on Chinese ideograms. The book of her poetry I printed in 1981. "*Plants would get most answers right / if left to themselves. / Seeds have good heads / given any luck at all. / And that moon tonight,/you watch it. / That moon and those trees / have worked together dividing things / since they were girls.*"

from *Dividing the Fields*

Crossing the border

Much of the language of cancer has to do with borders, with boundaries, with containment. The doctors don't really know the extent of cancer in my breast. Is it just one branch or many branches? It is important to make sure the cancer does not cross through the cell wall. I have spent the last twenty years breaking barriers and exploring new territory. How ironic to focus so fervently now on keeping within bounds.

with the main road. We are rarely here in this privileged zone of the front door, the drive, the stairs up to the heavy doors. Only on special occasions, such as fire drills. Our turf, a large square of playground to the side of the school. We usually come and go through side or back doors. Our tree, a grand tree with hollow large enough for us to enter, with gnarled roots. We race around it, chasing each other; other girls skip rope in another part of the yard, chanting jumping rhymes.

We are slightly beside ourselves at the novelty of manila paper, having drawing pencils, and being let out at this time of day. Yet we are expected to sit quietly and await further instruction. The ground is hard, with small rocks and roots making our exercise harder than it looks. Blades of grass leave sweaty green dents on our legs if we sit in one spot too long. I am seized with the desire to throw myself on the ground and stare up into the tree. We group tightly together and look up into the tree, but we are to draw it from a side view. I won't see a tree painted from underneath for fifteen more years, when I see O'Keeffe's painting of the Lawrence Tree. I don't actually see the painting, but see it in reproduction, first in black and white, and finally in color.

The radio oncologist draws me a picture of what has happened inside my breast. Tiny branches of cancer shoot out from a main branch of the milk ducts. He explains the clusters of cancer in my breast are tree-like, branching from the same stem.

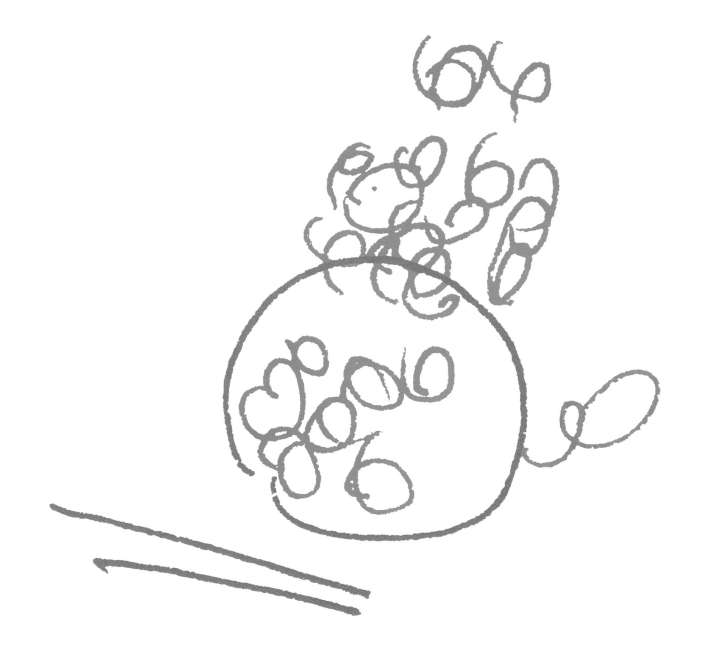

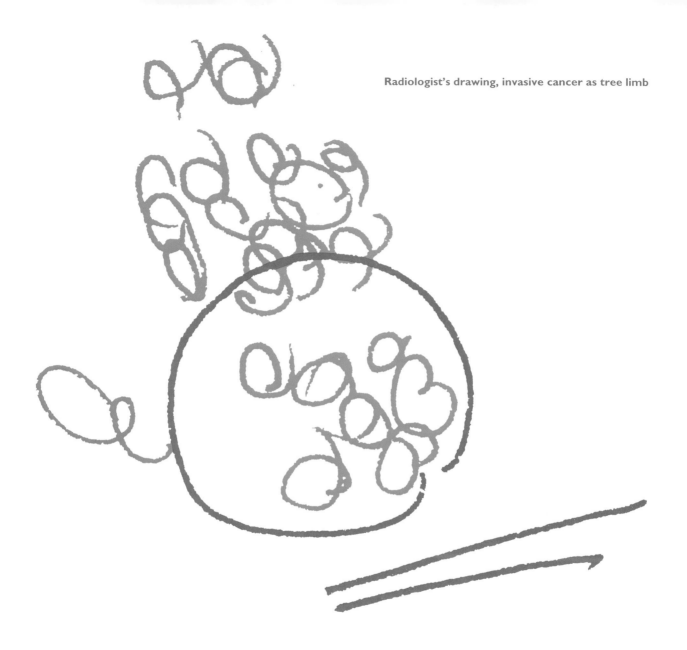

Radiologist's drawing, invasive cancer as tree limb

The proper way to draw a tree:

Use a pencil. Start with the trunk and draw it, starting near the bottom of the page. Now draw the other side. At about the middle of the page, make the lines farther apart. These are two limbs. Now draw the inside of each limb. IMPORTANT: Never let these limbs touch. Small limbs branch out from larger limbs. Small limbs branch into smaller limbs. Never let the lines touch. When you get to the smallest, tiniest limbs, leave the end of the limbs open.

The cancer cells are drawn differently from the unaffected area. The problem: These cells are still growing in the tunnels of my breasts. Or that is what they think. The important thing is that these cells don't cross over the duct wall, into the rest of my body. They must stay contained.

To properly paint leaves on a tree you need:
A Dixie cup full of yellow tempera paint
A Dixie cup full of blue tempera paint
Cotton swabs
Take a swab of yellow and place it over the swab of blue. In the right amounts, you will have green blobs that will be leaves.

Parking Lot Tree

Every weekday morning I validate my own parking receipt with a rubber stamp of a pine tree. The medical center is called Parkside, and there is a reminder, a remainder, a hint of grass, a green strip of grass that circles the parking lot. When did park become parking? The tree explanation of my doctor, the rubber stamp, the park turned to cement take on great significance. Everything is linked.

The Necklace

The museums were still disorganized by the war, and objects not properly labeled which slowed up my amateur investigation. But I worked my way back through the Bronze age to Neolithic figures. . . . One caught my eye. Three inches high, of sandy clay, a heavy-breasted little figure held a child, which was not more than a pinched blob of clay, crooked in her arm. I did not know from what part of the world she came, nor from what period. . . .

I visit Worpswede the way things happen on trips, a chance encounter opens to opportunity. The response to my question about interesting things to do in Germany comes as an echo, from unexpected quarters. It hasn't come from my friend, an artist who loves to travel, but from her friend standing beside her. They are both named Marian. Her friend, the unknown Marian, answers by asking if I wanted to "have a little travel adventure?" I listen with half an ear, not charmed by her coyness, and wondering if it was a trick question. But my curiosity is piqued. She unrolls a poster sent by a family friend, outlining a year-long celebration at a nearby artists' colony celebrating its 100th anniversary. With the poster comes an insistent invitation to visit Germany. The invitation, underlined like certain events on the calendar, seems more of a command than a request. Apparently someone has to show up. It might as well be me. She carefully explains to me the significance of the location, Worpswede, an artists' colony near Bremen in northern Germany. Its most famous resident, seventy-five years after its heyday, is Paula Modersohn-Becker, a painter. During the time I've planned to be in Germany, there will be a major exhibit of her work. Marian is so sure I had no knowledge of these names, that she says them slowly. And they do, here in the light of a bright Saturday in California, sound like names from another reality. My eyes widen. I know the names well.

Paula's destinations, from Bremen to Worpswede to Berlin to Worpswede to Paris and back again, loop around northern

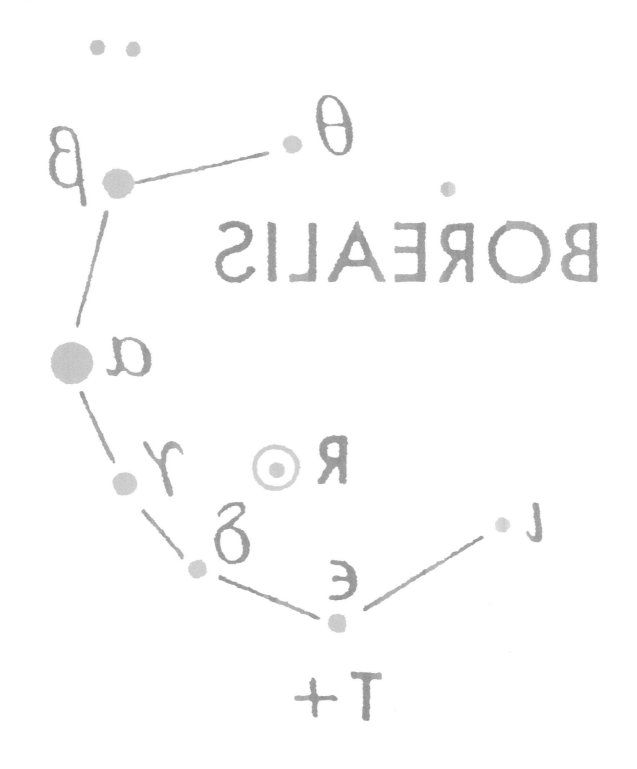

Ariadne helps Theseus
through the maze. She is
eventually turned into the
Corona Borealis.

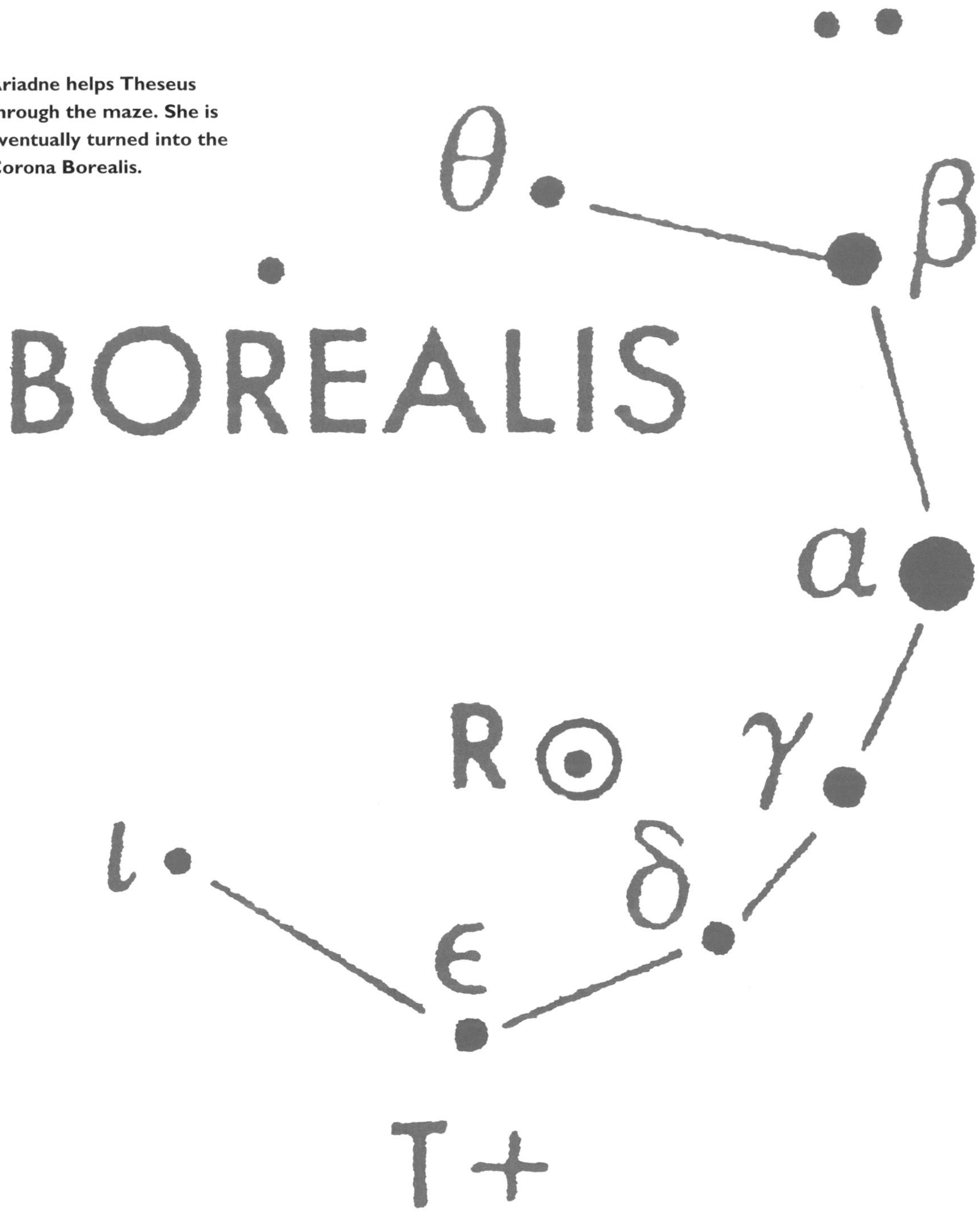

θ

β

BOREALIS

α

R ⊙

γ

ι

δ

ϵ

T +

Europe like beads on a string that become the story of her life. Her real destination is always Paris. From an early age, she buys time in the form of trips to Paris, stretching the weeks to months, staying as long as she can on each visit. First she travels to look at art, and then to paint. But she always returns to Worpswede, even under duress. It seems her true home, and her paintings show, I imagine, the influence of this remote village in northern Germany. I know these locales from her descriptions in letters written to parents, aunts, friends such as the poet Rilke, and later to her husband, the painter Otto Modersohn. I've spent two rainy winters reading about her life. Her descriptions give me the essence of places I never bother to look up on the map: I am sure I'll never go there, no matter how much I want to see these sites I've visited on the printed page. Instead, I find a slim volume of her paintings and see her life laid out in them: the young children and old women of Worpswede; the models drawn in the studios of Paris; the landscapes from unidentified locations; and finally, a remarkable series of seminude self-portraits, always with a flower or leaf in her hand, and a string of beads around her neck.

The month between the surgery and the start of radiation, I decide I need an amulet to help me survive the next phase of treatment. I find a necklace of blue glass beads at a wonderful bead store a block from my studio. I have many necklaces, most with curious old beads from the 1930s. They've been bought at flea markets around town and in other parts of the

. . . I did not know why her nose was like a bird—I did not know why, wearing nothing else, she should wear a necklace.
(This strange circumstance is widespread and I have not yet discovered the answer. Briffault refers to an Indian people who believe that her soul resides in a woman's necklace and she must not take it off. This question has remained strangely unexplored by anthropologists.)

Seonaid M. Robertson

**The Language
of the Goddess**

**Marija Gimbutas describes
beads in the shape of a
breast, the breasts of the
life-giving goddess. The
marks on the breast-shaped
beads, Vs and Xs and paral-
lel lines, look like surgery
scars. Gimbutas says they
are images of raindrops,
creeks, and streams of milk.**

country. They always remind me of middle European women
of a certain age. There is no time to search flea markets for
the right object, and my routine and route are getting smaller, my traveling more circumscribed. My choice is a choker,
something to wear on my body, close to my breast. It isn't too
long, it won't hang too low and interfere with my tender
scars. I've always had other problems with jewelry: the ten-
dency of bracelets to get in my way when I need my hands
free to work, or necklaces hanging too close to machinery. I
will wear the necklace and Rachel's angel every day, except
for my fifteen minutes every morning with the radiation
machines. For those few minutes I will have to disrobe from
the waist up. A seminude self-portrait without beads. The
only flower, the red rosettes of the lasers directed across my
body. I have some idea that the largest beads, the blue glass
ones, put on immediately following treatment, will absorb
and neutralize excess radiation, that their coolness will
soothe my skin, just burned by radium. And their deep blue
color is an important aspect, although I can't say how.

By wearing the beads, I take Paula with me. I need the
wholeness of her self-portraits. I need the strength of her
frontal nudity, her self-observation, the artist looking directly
at her own naked body, which I can barely manage now. As
the days and weeks of radiation burn my body, I don't recog-
nize myself. Most of the artist's bodies I've seen in the last
decade have been the self-mutilated and tortured bodies of
performance artists in grainy black-and-white photos. I don't

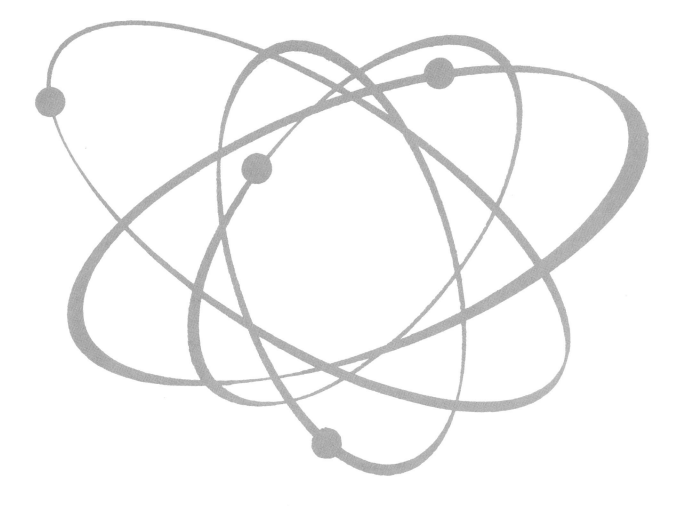

Atomic necklace
My drawing, sculpture L.A. County Art Museum

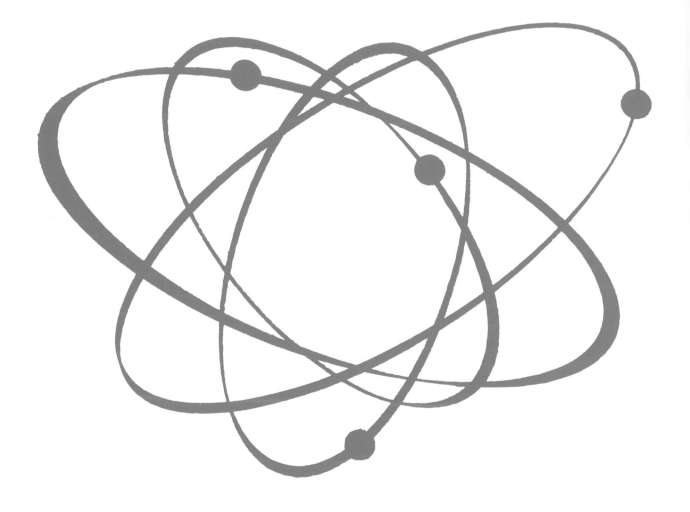

need to see more of that. I need her healthiness, her sense of well-being. My right breast hasn't been this small since I was in high school. I need to see her body, another woman's body, an artist's body, relaxed, not on alert as my breast becomes hardened, changed and burned by the treatments of radium administered daily.

As the surgeon unwraps my breast, a scene from some old movie flashes across my brain. Bette Davis, someone, is having bandages removed from her head and her eyes. In a moment she will know if she is permanently blind. I've just been told there was no more cancer found, but it is this moment, the unwrapping of the breast, that is the real moment of truth for me. My breast looks pale and shrunken, as if it's been underwater for the last three days. Traumatized but still there, at least part of it is still there. I am deliriously happy about my prognosis, and exhausted by everything I've had to endure.

Finally, I leave the hospital and come back home.

In between sleeping and taking synthetic narcotics I read Edna O'Brien's novels in the week after I've come home from the hospital. I follow Kate and Baba through Ireland, through entire lives in *The Country Girls Trilogy and Epilogue* and then coax Mike to go to library to get *A Fanatic Heart*. We go to Santa Barbara for a weekend away from the radiation treatments; I sleep most of the weekend but on one of our few

Art I see on the medical pilgrimage:

Jaime's pastels of Norway in the waiting room of the surgeon.

Watercolors of the beach at the radiologist's office.

Bonnard poster with yellow pigments bleached out at internist's examining room.

Van Gogh's *Irises* poster in the hallway of the plastic surgeon's office . . .

. . . A Cast paper *drawing* in the examining room of the plastic surgeon makes me nervous. It is not real art. It is art made for corporate offices such as these, or perhaps it is art made by a family member, friend, or patient of the doctor. It has glitter and a crayon gash.

outings I manage to find an out-of-print collection of her short stories at a used bookstore there. Mike finds her writing depressing. I find her emotion-filled novels a balm during my convalescence.

As soon as I can drive again, I drive myself to daily bargain matinees. My own treatment has been to wander the museums. Go to the movies. At one point, I have seen eleven of the movies at the fourteen-screen theater near the studio, a record I'd never achieve in my normally busy life. I wander aimlessly through the museum late on weekday mornings. I discover whole rooms, whole floors of art I never knew existed. Art and movies become a salvation. I stand before paintings, before sculptures of Indian deities, sit in darkened theaters and lose myself for a few hours. But my time is limited and turned around. By 4:30, my witching hour, I must be home, near the futon in my loft. The radiation absorbs all my late-afternoon energy. This used to be my favorite time of day. Now I am useless. It is all I can do to drag myself to bed. Then I'm up again, at three in the morning, watching old movies on all-night TV.

I still live close to Hollywood. Even though I've had cancer, Hollywood, and the rest of the world, is unchanged. And life imitates art, or what passes for art here in L.A. On my first visit to a cancer support group, the woman registering us at the orientation meeting announces, breathlessly, that the

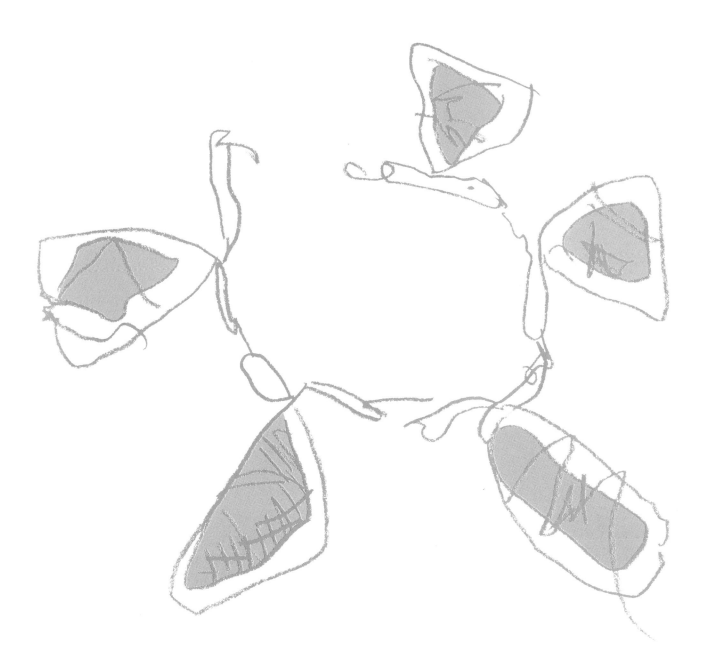

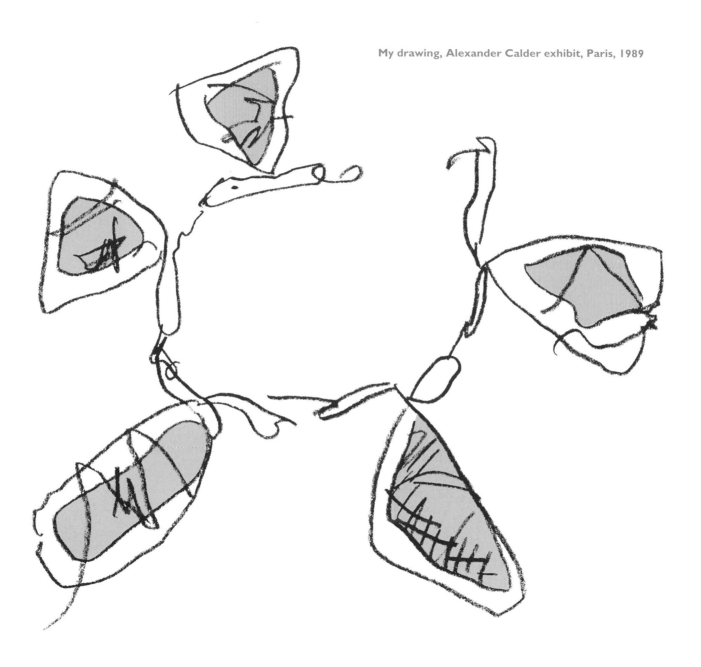

My drawing, Alexander Calder exhibit, Paris, 1989

center will be part of an upcoming TV show, part of *thirtysomething*, the yuppie drama I've been watching with renewed interest since both Nancy, one of the main characters, and I have cancer. The receptionist assumes we'll all feel validated by having our disease written into a TV show. And it will be taped here, this very week, a support group just like this one. Cancer on TV is more exciting, more vivid, more dramatic than what we are going through. It only takes up one hour a week. And if you're not up to dealing with it, it can be turned off with a flick of the remote control.

When the support group episode airs, I am cautiously optimistic as I watch a middle-aged free spirit at the cancer group start to wake Nancy up. Nancy goes wild, doing irrational, spontaneous things she hasn't allowed herself since art school. This extreme shift of consciousness lasts until the break in the middle of the show. Something happens during the three commercials that we don't see on screen. When we return to the show, the free spirit's cancer wig comes off. She is really a cancer witch. Nancy comes to her senses (or doesn't, depending on your view) in the nick of time. She knuckles under, returns to sacrificing herself to her family. Her biggest sacrifice: to ditch a breakthrough in her art and make a children's book with her son. I scream at the TV. I have watched this for weeks! Weeks! Even in the hospital. How dare they make this the ending? I will write a letter to the show. I compose it for the next two weeks in my head. But the truth is, I need my energy for something else, for everything else.

Postscript

As I finish up work on this book: I undergo a second biopsy. The tissue removed from my other breast is benign.

I hear the following statistics: In America a woman dies of breast cancer every eleven minutes.

I read, in a newsletter for women photographers, that Jo Spence died in 1992 of lymphatic leukemia.

By the most desperate and arid effort they discovered a magic element, radium. I sit in the radiologist's office and read a sentimental biography of Madame Curie. I grow tired of the writing and change to the cool and distant story of the haiku poet Basho and his trip to the Far North in May 1689. He was forty-five years old, and was on the road for five months. He didn't expect to return alive.

The Afterword/Afterward

Seven years ago this month I fashioned a sabbatical for myself and flew to Amsterdam to begin the first part of the journey described here. As the text reveals, it was more of an adventure than I'd planned. I couldn't have known that my trip would be bounded by breast cancer: my mother's mastectomy as I arrived in Amsterdam, my book dealer's death in London from metastasized breast cancer, and my own diagnosis and treatment the following winter. Yet time has given me the luxury of being a "maze viewer who sees the pattern whole." Time, and early diagnosis and treatment. So, after being inextricably bound to walk the labyrinth, often not knowing what lay around the next turn, I'm now able to see the complex artistry in my own situation, something not possible while I was traveling through medieval Europe or on the road of illness here in Los Angeles.

In America, many of our stories end in a linear fashion: happily every after on the other side of a picket fence, or here in the West, a ride into the sunset to the strains of "Happy Trails to You." My journey didn't end with a destination reached. My journey continues—forever part of a cycle. The circle just gets bigger as I walk out of the labyrinth.

Two years after my treatment, one of my doctors declared me cured. I finally felt able to put down these stories in the form I know best, a book. Writing this book was a chance to look at and re-experience these journeys. I'd been aware of certain images during my trip that loomed large during my

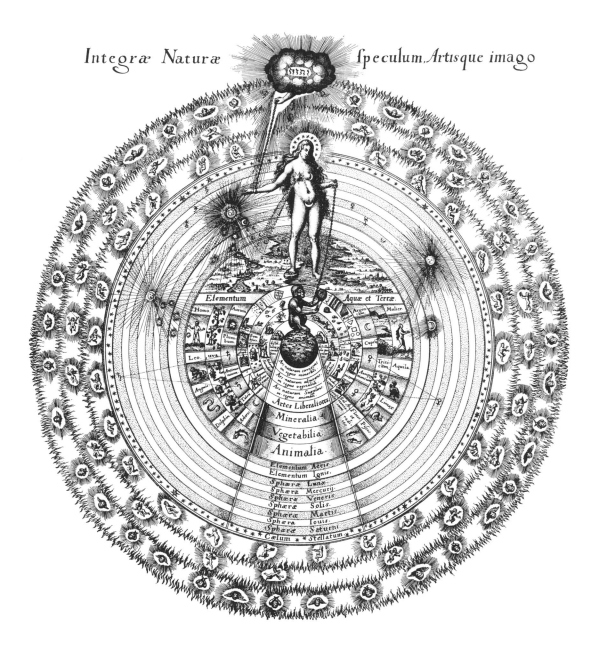

Integræ Naturæ *Speculum, Artisque imago*

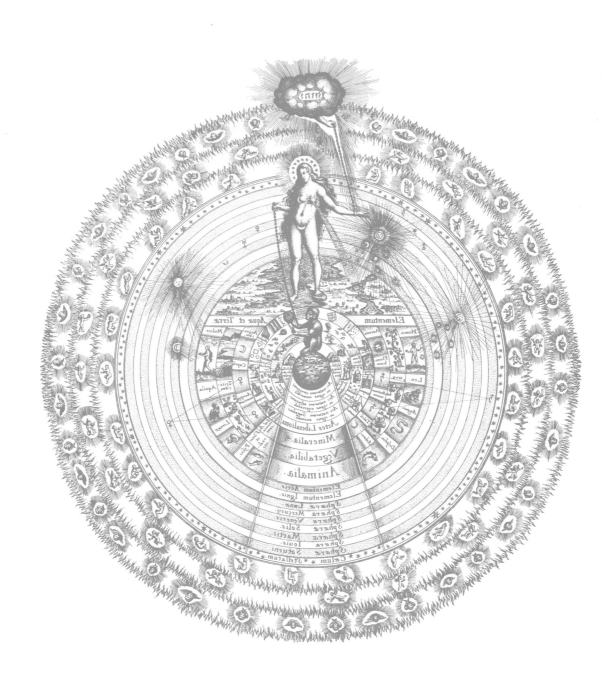

illness. I finally had time to discover the connection between the pattern of the tiny red lasers used in radiation therapy and the pattern of the rose window at Chartres Cathedral, both healing mandalas separated by ages and radically different ways of looking at the world. I wanted time to think about the ways in which both trips were similar. The isolation and silence I'd felt traveling alone was mirrored in the isolation of illness. It seemed impossible to investigate these connections in the midst of treatment. My attention had been on survival and getting well. Now I felt ready, but it was still tender territory. I began slowly.

Support was forthcoming from Montage, a citywide festival in Rochester, New York. I was one of three artists chosen to produce the first edition of a book at Visual Studies Workshop, an art center in Rochester that helps artists produce visual books. With their support I knew the project would get made. In the middle of preparing the artwork and text for the printer, I underwent a second biopsy. Suddenly I was back in the spiral of illness again. In some ways it was worse the second time. The biopsy turned out benign, but I was left with the realization that I would never truly be free of this in my life. There will always be the possibility of reoccurrence of breast cancer.

I sat at my computer just about every day that winter and retraced my steps. Some of it was exceedingly hard. It took me a week to take some negatives of self-portraits I'd done before and after my biopsy and surgery to be made into

The Sabbatical implies leaving a field fallow on the seventh year or resting on the Sabbath — the seventh day in some religions. Today the sabbatical means a release from normal duties, a chance to step back from everyday life and take a deep breath, to do something entirely different for a calendar year, with the idea of returning to the same job, the same circumstance a changed person, or at least a refreshed one.

prints. I could hardly stand to look at the proof sheets again. Other tasks were easier: I looked at postcards of medieval books, scraps of ephemera I'd collected along the way, and re-read my travel diary. I looked at every piece of paper in my medical file. I loved being in the earlier stages of research, surrounded by a pile of books, following some illogical train of thought I knew not where. I found I could fill whole mornings that way. The connections I was making were exciting. Each piece of writing was read by my writer's group, where it was critically reviewed. Their comments helped me shape it. I traveled to Rochester and worked there for a month, living at the art center and working on my book every day and lots of nights. I worked right through a blizzard that paralyzed the East Coast. As always, making art out of my experience helped transform it. Each step in production helped me release the experience and some of the agony of treatment. I re-assumed the role of artist, rather than patient.

Marian Winsryg, an artist here in L.A., recently curated an exhibit called "One in Eight: Women and Breast Cancer." Talking to her was helpful. I had doubts about placing highly personal work in public view. Once people know I've had cancer, will they treat me differently? When I expressed this to her, she turned to me and said bluntly" Face it. You *are* different." Her words were more accurate than she could know.

If you live in your body, you face a lot. I'd already faced the surgeon's knife. I'd faced a spring of radiation treatments and prolonged fatigue. It appeared I'd made a miraculous recovery only to encounter profound grief a year after my treatment. I was happy to be alive, but I suddenly felt a tremendous sense of loss. My doctor had no solution. Once again it was up to me. I contacted a therapist I'd seen a few years before and talked to him. I muddled along. Doing the best I could to deal with each new thing I encountered on the path. Treading the Maze.

The response to my illness has been varied. I have friends who continue to be there for me, all these years later. I have friends that act as if it never happened, some have told me, because they don't know what to say. Yet I've received effusive response to this book from complete strangers who've gone through the experience themselves, or whose best friend, sister, mother, or aunt are going through the experience now. Often they want another copy to be sent as a gift.

I get calls from friends telling me of scores of people with the disease. Sometimes I can help. I tell them what's been helpful to me: Stay in touch even if you don't know what to say or do; illness can be extremely isolating. Offer to do one thing for the person. It could be as simple as picking up books from the library, or making a trip to the grocery. If its someone I am very close to, and the person is going through a critical time, my husband or I call everyday.

Sometimes I can't bear to hear another story about illness. On these days I do something that was difficult before my illness. I practice compassion, this time towards myself. I remind myself that it's OK to just listen and not do anything.

Bibliography

John Adair, *The Pilgrim's Way.* Thames and Hudson, 1978.

Eve Curie, *Madame Curie.* Doubleday, Doran & Company, 1937.

Mary Daly, *Websters' First New Intergalactic Wickedary of the English Language.* Beacon Press, 1987.

Penelope Reed Doob, *The Idea of the Labyrinth.* Cornell University Press, 1990.

Lesley Downer. *On The Narrow Road: Journey into a Lost Japan.* Summit Books, 1989.

Clarissa Pinkola Estes, *Women Who Run with the Wolves.* Ballantine Books, 1992.

Marija Gimbutas, *The Language of the Goddess.* Harper and Row, 1989.

Eloise Klein Healy, *Ordinary Wisdom.* Paradise Press, 1981.

James Joyce, *Dubliners.* Modern Library, 1967.

Lucy R. Lippard, *Overlay: Contemporary Art and the Art of Prehistory.* Pantheon Books, 1983.

Seonaid M. Robertson, *Rosegarden and Labyrinth.* Spring Publications, 1982.

Jo Spence, *Putting Myself in the Picture.* Camden Press, 1986.

Laurens Van der Post, *Venture to the Interior.* Morrow, 1951.

I never had problems knowing I was stressed; the difference is now I heed the warning signs. I've continued my own regime of treatment: bodywork to help counter the fatigue and stress my body had been through, more relaxation, and a real change in the way I deal with stress at work. I find myself less willing to put up with intolerable situations.

Friends tell me all sort of stories of recovery. One artist had come back with a roar, works harder than ever, and seems unstoppable. Another woman barely skips a beat; she had a mastectomy and was back at work as soon as possible. I've chosen another path, I think. One that has me circling this illness, thinking about it, writing about it. Not ignoring its meaning or significance.

I still do many of the things I've always done: make artist's books, do the chores, spend time with my husband and pet the cat. Whole days go by and I don't think about cancer. I can tell things have changed when I talk about my work. Every time I give a slide presentation, I know *this* piece is coming, lurking, at the end of my talk. My artwork is not particularly frivolous, but it does contain a lot of humor. I know when I start talking about "this book I've made about my journey through cancer" there will suddenly be complete silence in the hall. Its as if a large presence has walked into the room and left us in a state of awe. And I stand there in the dark, and read from my book one more time, words still so close to my heart. I feel the story drop as I read, drop to a deeper level—into the Land of Cancer. I read the piece about waiting: "Waiting for news of the biopsy. . . .waiting for someone in the recovery room to pull a blanket up over my knees . . . .waiting to be next in line for radiation therapy." Sometimes I can't catch my breath. I'm back in the experience in a second. And I just take a deep breath and go on.

Barbara G. Walker, *The Woman's Encyclopedia of Myths and Secrets*. Harper and Row, 1983.

Hebe 1806 is a marble sculpture by Bertel Thorvaldsen. Used with permission, Thorvaldsen's Museum, Copenhagen. Photo by Ole Woldbye

Acknowledgments

Many people have walked parts of the maze with me. Early drafts of this book were read by Bonnie Barrett, Nora Dvosin, Ann Glover, Michele Kort, Maureen Murdock, and Aleida Rodriguez. Allwynn O'Mara's generous spirit and her skill with book structures were critical in the design stage of the first edition. Joan and Nathan Lyons at Visual Studies Workshop helped make the first edition a reality. Joan was project director for my book as well. Paul Muhly, the printer at vsw, took extra care with the presswork. His experience and good nature made the making of the first edition a pleasure. Special thanks to Montage International Festival of the Image, 1993, for publishing the first edition.

Doctors Phyllis Klein, Michael Steinberg and Ruth Carr helped me through the medical maze of my illness. Dr. Barbara Rapko, RN, and acupressure practitioner bridged the worlds of Eastern and Western medicine. She and Dr. Barry Mann are gifted healers and I feel blessed to have had them in my life during this period.

Thanks to Mary Daly, Lesley Downer, Seonaid M. Robertson, Jo Spence, Lucy Lippard and the poet Basho whose writings inspired me, and to Bertel Thorvaldsen whose sculpture spoke to me through time and space. Catherine Horton, Pat Robertson and Terry Braunstein know about keeping images alive. Their creative minds and hearts fostered the project at many stages.

Gary Chassman at Verve Editions gave the book a second life. His vision, faith and hard work have been remarkable. Thanks to Wynne Patterson for her design. Her sensitivity to the spirit of the original is more than I could have hoped. Thanks to Carolyn Herter at Chronicle Books who steered the project with care through to publication and into the world.

Lastly, thanks to Michael Oppenheim and Rachel Barclay. They support my life and work in ways trivial and great.

**Cathedral de Chartres
Labyrinth © E Houvet**

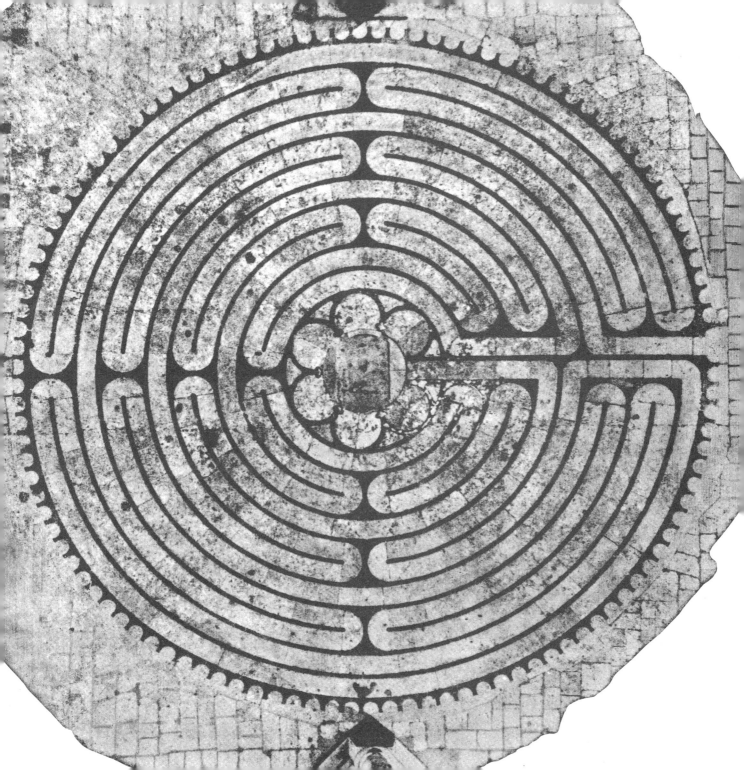

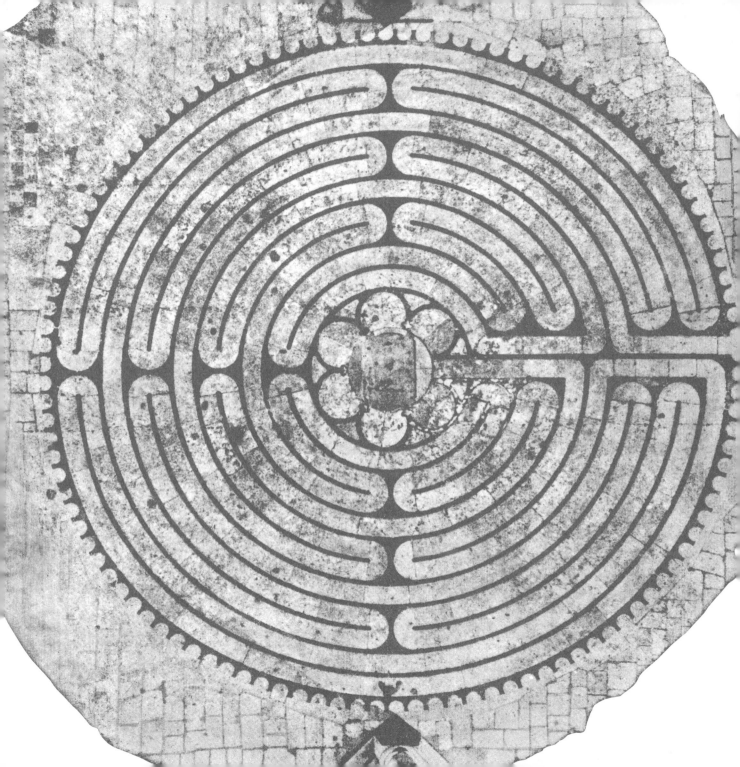